FOCUS ON FITNESS NOT THINNESS WORKBOOK

HAYLEY CANOVA

Copyright © 2025 Utah Publishing, LLC.

All rights reserved. No portion of this book may be reproduced or transmitted in any form or by any means without written permission from the author or publisher.

ISBN: 979-8-9985202-3-5

MEDICAL AND LEGAL DISCLAIMER
The information contained herein is intended solely for educational and informational purposes and should not be relied upon as medical advice or to replace the advice of a qualified healthcare professional. The author is not a licensed healthcare provider and the information in this book should not be considered a substitute for professional medical advice regarding prevention, diagnosis, or treatment of disease.

The author has made every effort to ensure that the information provided in this book is accurate and up-to-date. However, neither the author nor publishing company make representations or warranties of any kind, express or implied, about the completeness, accuracy, reliability, suitability, or availability, with respect to the information contained in this book. Neither the author nor publishing company shall be liable for any loss, injury, or damages, including but not limited to any direct, indirect, consequential, or incidental damages nor losses arising out of or in connection with the use, reliance, or inability to use the information in this book.

The reader should consult with a licensed healthcare professional before undertaking any new nutrition plan, exercise program, or wellness program, or before making any changes to their current healthcare regimen. The reader should not disregard professional medical advice or delay seeking it because of information provided in this book.

The author and publishing company disclaim any responsibility for any actions taken by the reader, based on the information provided in this book.

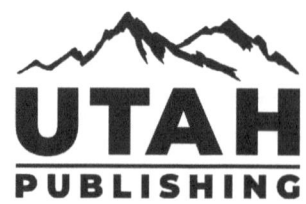

For additional healthy recipes and basic exercise tutorials, please find me on YouTube, Instagram, TikTok, or Facebook. Follow, like, or subscribe so that you never miss a post! Thank you!

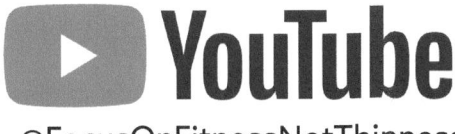
@FocusOnFitnessNotThinness

HealthyByHay

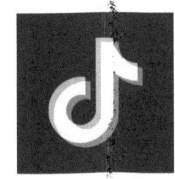
@healthy.by.hay

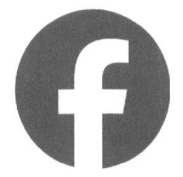
Healthy By Hay

MEAL PLANNER

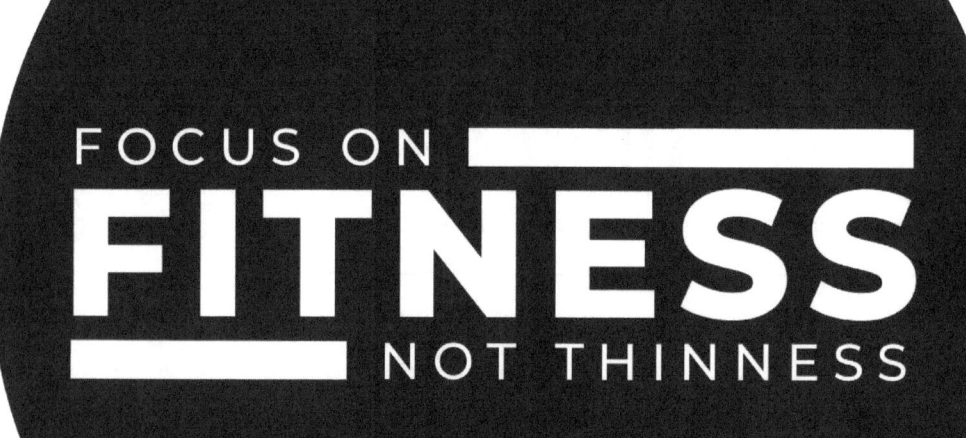

FOCUS ON
FITNESS
NOT THINNESS

MY MEAL PLANS

MEAL PLANNER

MEAL PLAN (VARIETY)

		SUN	MON	TUE	WED	THU	FRI	SAT
WEEK 1	BREAKFAST	AVOCADO TOAST	ALMOND TOAST	FRUIT & OATS BOWL	CHOCOLATE PB SHAKE	AVOCADO TOAST	ALMOND TOAST	BANANA SHAKE
	LUNCH	CHICKEN NUGGETS	PECAN SALAD	GR CHICKEN SALAD	SNACK WRAPS	RANCH POTATO	PECAN SALAD	CRISPY BEAN BURRITOS
	DINNER	BAKED SALMON	BAKED FAJITAS	ALMOND CHICKEN	KUNG PAO CHICKEN	LETTUCE WRAPS	SESAME CHICKEN	HONEY LIME FLAUTAS
WEEK 2	BREAKFAST	AVOCADO TOAST	ALMOND TOAST	FRUIT & OATS BOWL	CHOCOLATE PB SHAKE	AVOCADO TOAST	ALMOND TOAST	BANANA SHAKE
	LUNCH	CHICKEN NUGGETS	RANCH POTATO	PECAN SALAD	SNACK WRAPS	GR CHICKEN SALAD	PECAN SALAD	CRISPY BEAN BURRITOS
	DINNER	SWEET PORK SALAD	SOUTHWEST SALAD	ORANGE CHICKEN	CRISPY CHK SALAD	WRAPPED TOSTADA	CHICKEN PARMESAN	ST LOUIS BOWL
WEEK 3	BREAKFAST	AVOCADO TOAST	ALMOND TOAST	FRUIT & OATS BOWL	CHOCOLATE PB SHAKE	AVOCADO TOAST	ALMOND TOAST	BANANA SHAKE
	LUNCH	CHICKEN NUGGETS	RANCH POTATO	PECAN SALAD	SNACK WRAPS	GR CHICKEN SALAD	CRISPY BEAN BURRITOS	PECAN SALAD
	DINNER	SALMON SUSHI BOWL	HAWAIIAN PLATE	GREEK GYROS	ELOTE TACOS	MANICOTTI	ALMOND CHICKEN	PINEAPPLE KABOBS
WEEK 4	BREAKFAST	AVOCADO TOAST	ALMOND TOAST	FRUIT & OATS BOWL	CHOCOLATE PB SHAKE	AVOCADO TOAST	ALMOND TOAST	BANANA SHAKE
	LUNCH	CHICKEN NUGGETS	SNACK WRAPS	RANCH POTATO	PECAN SALAD	CRISPY BEAN BURRITOS	SNACK WRAPS	GR CHICKEN SALAD
	DINNER	BARBACOA BURRITO	TERIYAKI BOWL	POLLO ASADO	HONEY LIME FLAUTAS	LETTUCE WRAPS	ORANGE CHICKEN	CHICKEN PARMESAN
WEEK 5	BREAKFAST	ALMOND TOAST	FRUIT & OATS BOWL	CHOCOLATE PB SHAKE	AVOCADO TOAST	ALMOND TOAST	BANANA SHAKE	AVOCADO TOAST
	LUNCH	RANCH POTATO	PECAN SALAD	SNACK WRAPS	GR CHICKEN SALAD	CRISPY BEAN BURRITOS	SNACK WRAPS	CHICKEN NUGGETS
	DINNER	ST LOUIS BOWL	CRISPY CHK SALAD	SWT POTATO CURRY	FISH TACOS	WRAPPED TOSTADA	PINEAPPLE KABOBS	BAKED SALMON

MEAL PLANNER

MEAL PLAN (PRACTICAL)

	SUN	MON	TUE	WED	THU	FRI	SAT
WEEK 1 BREAKFAST	ALMOND TOAST	BANANA SHAKE	FRUIT & OATS BOWL	CHOCOLATE PB SHAKE	ALMOND TOAST	AVOCADO TOAST	FRUIT & OATS BOWL
LUNCH	PECAN SALAD	SNACK WRAPS	RANCH POTATO	DINNER LEFTOVERS	GR CHICKEN SALAD	CRISPY BEAN BURRITOS	RANCH POTATO
DINNER	LETTUCE WRAPS	CHICKEN PARMESAN	GREEK GYROS	BAKED SALMON	ALMOND CHICKEN	SESAME CHICKEN	HONEY LIME FLAUTAS
WEEK 2 BREAKFAST	ALMOND TOAST	FRUIT & OATS BOWL	AVOCADO TOAST	BANANA SHAKE	FRUIT & OATS BOWL	CHOCOLATE PB SHAKE	FRUIT & OATS BOWL
LUNCH	BARBACOA BURRITO	SOUTHWEST SALAD	ORANGE CHICKEN	RANCH POTATO	KUNG PAO CHICKEN	PECAN SALAD	ST LOUIS BOWL
DINNER	DINNER LEFTOVERS	DINNER LEFTOVERS	MANICOTTI	DINNER LEFTOVERS	DINNER LEFTOVERS	POLLO ASADO	DINNER LEFTOVERS
WEEK 3 BREAKFAST	ALMOND TOAST	BANANA SHAKE	ALMOND TOAST	AVOCADO TOAST	ALMOND TOAST	CHOCOLATE PB SHAKE	FRUIT & OATS BOWL
LUNCH	HAWAIIAN PLATE	WRAPPED TOSTADA	PECAN SALAD	SNACK WRAPS	GR CHICKEN SALAD	PECAN SALAD	BAKED FAJITAS
DINNER	DINNER LEFTOVERS	DINNER LEFTOVERS	DINNER LEFTOVERS	TERIYAKI BOWL	ELOTE TACOS	DINNER LEFTOVERS	SWT POTATO CURRY
WEEK 4 BREAKFAST	ALMOND TOAST	BANANA SHAKE	AVOCADO TOAST	CHOCOLATE PB SHAKE	ALMOND TOAST	AVOCADO TOAST	FRUIT & OATS BOWL
LUNCH	SNACK WRAPS	DINNER LEFTOVERS	CHICKEN NUGGETS	RANCH POTATO	PECAN SALAD	DINNER LEFTOVERS	DINNER LEFTOVERS
DINNER	SWEET PORK SALAD	CRISPY CHK SALAD	SESAME CHICKEN	CHICKEN PARMESAN	LETTUCE WRAPS	SALMON SUSHI BOWL	CRISPY BEAN BURRITOS
WEEK 5 BREAKFAST	AVOCADO TOAST	AVOCADO TOAST	BANANA SHAKE	FRUIT & OAT BOWL	ALMOND TOAST	CHOCOLATE PB SHAKE	FRUIT & OATS BOWL
LUNCH	GR CHICKEN SALAD	DINNER LEFTOVERS	CHICKEN NUGGETS	DINNER LEFTOVERS	PECAN SALAD	DINNER LEFTOVERS	DINNER LEFTOVERS
DINNER	KUNG PAO CHICKEN	CRISPY CHK SALAD	GREEK GYROS	ALMOND CHICKEN	WRAPPED TOSTADA	SOUTHWEST SALAD	FISH TACOS

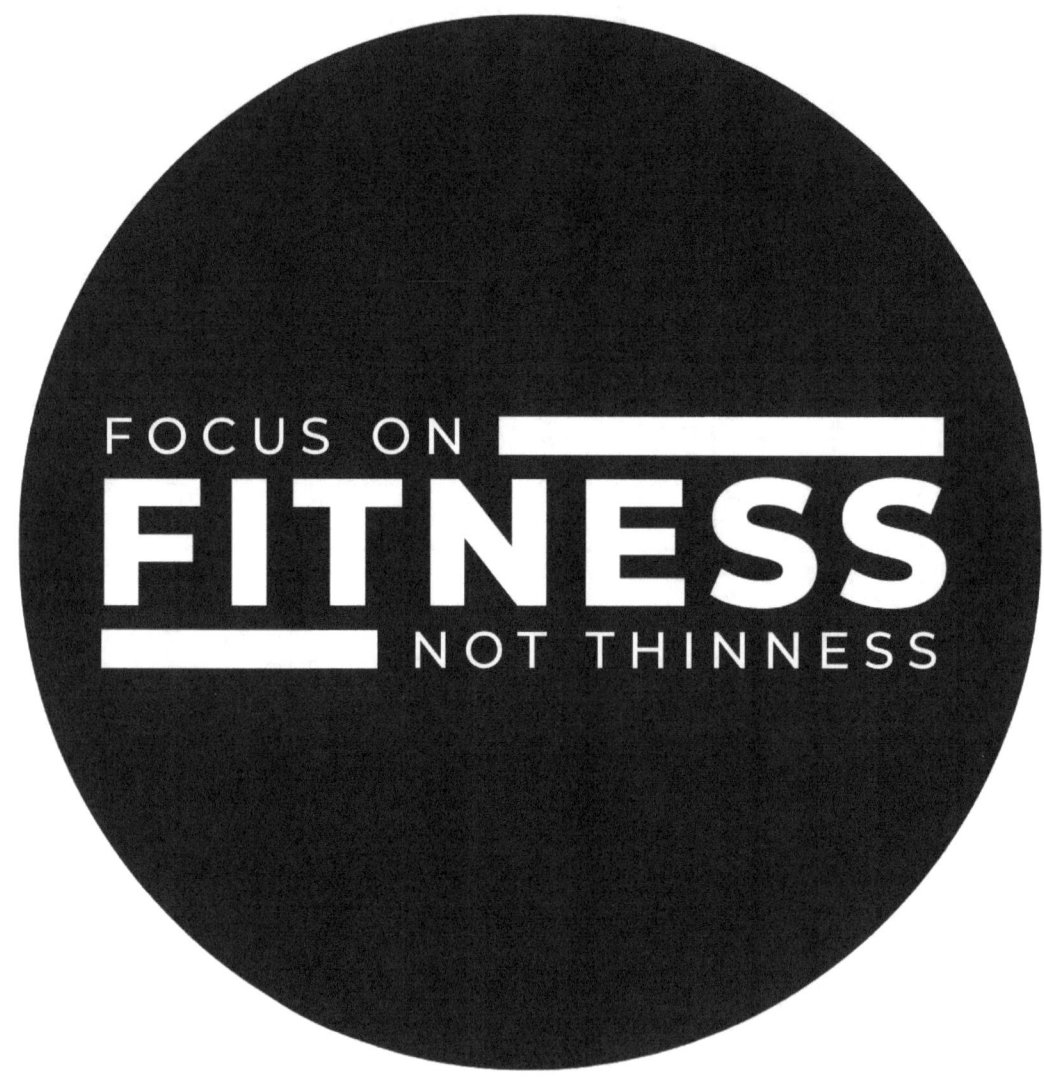

MY WORKOUT PLANS

WORKOUT PLANS

JUST GET MOVING PLAN

12-WEEK WORKOUT SCHEDULE

	SUN	MON	TUE	WED	THU	FRI	SAT
1	REST	15 MIN CARDIO	REST	15 MIN CARDIO	REST	15 MIN CARDIO	REST
2	REST	15 MIN CARDIO	REST	15 MIN CARDIO	REST	15 MIN CARDIO	REST
3	REST	15 MIN CARDIO	REST	15 MIN CARDIO	REST	15 MIN CARDIO	REST
4	REST	20 MIN CARDIO	REST	20 MIN CARDIO	REST	20 MIN CARDIO	REST
5	REST	20 MIN CARDIO	REST	20 MIN CARDIO	REST	20 MIN CARDIO	REST
6	REST	20 MIN CARDIO	REST	20 MIN CARDIO	REST	20 MIN CARDIO	REST
7	REST	25 MIN CARDIO	REST	25 MIN CARDIO	REST	25 MIN CARDIO	REST
8	REST	25 MIN CARDIO	REST	25 MIN CARDIO	REST	25 MIN CARDIO	REST
9	REST	25 MIN CARDIO	REST	25 MIN CARDIO	REST	25 MIN CARDIO	REST
10	REST	30 MIN CARDIO	REST	30 MIN CARDIO	REST	30 MIN CARDIO	REST
11	REST	30 MIN CARDIO	REST	30 MIN CARDIO	REST	30 MIN CARDIO	REST
12	REST	30 MIN CARDIO	REST	30 MIN CARDIO	REST	30 MIN CARDIO	REST

WORKOUT PLANS

BRONZE PLAN
12-WEEK WORKOUT SCHEDULE

	SUN	MON	TUE	WED	THU	FRI	SAT
1	REST	15 MIN CARDIO & 1 UPPER SET	REST	15 MIN CARDIO & 1 LOWER SET	REST	30 MIN CARDIO & 1 CORE SET	REST
2	REST	15 MIN CARDIO & 1 UPPER SET	REST	15 MIN CARDIO & 1 LOWER SET	REST	30 MIN CARDIO & 1 CORE SET	REST
3	REST	15 MIN CARDIO & 1 UPPER SET	REST	15 MIN CARDIO & 1 LOWER SET	REST	30 MIN CARDIO & 1 CORE SET	REST
4	REST	15 MIN CARDIO & 1 UPPER SET	REST	15 MIN CARDIO & 1 LOWER SET	REST	30 MIN CARDIO & 1 CORE SET	REST
5	REST	15 MIN CARDIO & 2 UPPER SET	REST	15 MIN CARDIO & 2 LOWER SET	REST	30 MIN CARDIO & 1 CORE SET	REST
6	REST	15 MIN CARDIO & 2 UPPER SET	REST	15 MIN CARDIO & 2 LOWER SET	REST	30 MIN CARDIO & 1 CORE SET	REST
7	REST	15 MIN CARDIO & 2 UPPER SET	REST	15 MIN CARDIO & 2 LOWER SET	REST	30 MIN CARDIO & 1 CORE SET	REST
8	REST	15 MIN CARDIO & 2 UPPER SET	REST	15 MIN CARDIO & 2 LOWER SET	REST	30 MIN CARDIO & 1 CORE SET	REST
9	REST	15 MIN CARDIO & 2 UPPER SET	REST	15 MIN CARDIO & 2 LOWER SET	REST	30 MIN CARDIO & 1 CORE SET	REST
10	REST	15 MIN CARDIO & 2 UPPER SET	REST	15 MIN CARDIO & 2 LOWER SET	REST	30 MIN CARDIO & 1 CORE SET	REST
11	REST	15 MIN CARDIO & 2 UPPER SET	REST	15 MIN CARDIO & 2 LOWER SET	REST	30 MIN CARDIO & 1 CORE SET	REST
12	REST	15 MIN CARDIO & 2 UPPER SET	REST	15 MIN CARDIO & 2 LOWER SET	REST	30 MIN CARDIO & 1 CORE SET	REST

WORKOUT PLANS

SILVER PLAN

12-WEEK WORKOUT SCHEDULE

	SUN	MON	TUE	WED	THU	FRI	SAT
1	REST	UPPER BODY 2 SETS	30 MIN CARDIO	REST	LOWER BODY 2 SETS	30 MIN CARDIO & 1 CORE SET	REST
2	REST	UPPER BODY 2 SETS	30 MIN CARDIO	REST	LOWER BODY 2 SETS	30 MIN CARDIO & 1 CORE SET	REST
3	REST	UPPER BODY 2 SETS	30 MIN CARDIO	REST	LOWER BODY 2 SETS	30 MIN CARDIO & 1 CORE SET	REST
4	REST	UPPER BODY 2 SETS	30 MIN CARDIO	REST	LOWER BODY 2 SETS	30 MIN CARDIO & 1 CORE SET	REST
5	REST	UPPER BODY 3 SETS	30 MIN CARDIO	REST	LOWER BODY 3 SETS	30 MIN CARDIO & 1 CORE SET	REST
6	REST	UPPER BODY 3 SETS	30 MIN CARDIO	REST	LOWER BODY 3 SETS	30 MIN CARDIO & 1 CORE SET	REST
7	REST	UPPER BODY 3 SETS	30 MIN CARDIO	REST	LOWER BODY 3 SETS	30 MIN CARDIO & 1 CORE SET	REST
8	REST	UPPER BODY 3 SETS	30 MIN CARDIO	REST	LOWER BODY 3 SETS	30 MIN CARDIO & 1 CORE SET	REST
9	REST	UPPER BODY 3 SETS	30 MIN CARDIO	REST	LOWER BODY 3 SETS	30 MIN CARDIO & 1 CORE SET	REST
10	REST	UPPER BODY 3 SETS	30 MIN CARDIO	REST	LOWER BODY 3 SETS	30 MIN CARDIO & 1 CORE SET	REST
11	REST	UPPER BODY 3 SETS	30 MIN CARDIO	REST	LOWER BODY 3 SETS	30 MIN CARDIO & 1 CORE SET	REST
12	REST	UPPER BODY 3 SETS	30 MIN CARDIO	REST	LOWER BODY 3 SETS	30 MIN CARDIO & 1 CORE SET	REST

WORKOUT PLANS

GOLD PLAN

12-WEEK WORKOUT SCHEDULE

	SUN	MON	TUE	WED	THU	FRI	SAT
1	REST	UPPER BODY 3 SETS	30 MIN CARDIO	LOWER BODY 3 SETS	30 MIN CARDIO	REST	15 MIN CARDIO & 1 CORE SET
2	REST	UPPER BODY 3 SETS	30 MIN CARDIO	LOWER BODY 3 SETS	30 MIN CARDIO	REST	15 MIN CARDIO & 1 CORE SET
3	REST	UPPER BODY 3 SETS	30 MIN CARDIO	LOWER BODY 3 SETS	30 MIN CARDIO	REST	15 MIN CARDIO & 1 CORE SET
4	REST	UPPER BODY 3 SETS	30 MIN CARDIO	LOWER BODY 3 SETS	30 MIN CARDIO	REST	15 MIN CARDIO & 1 CORE SET
5	REST	UPPER BODY 3 SETS	30 MIN CARDIO	LOWER BODY 3 SETS	30 MIN CARDIO	REST	15 MIN CARDIO & 1 CORE SET
6	REST	UPPER BODY 3 SETS	30 MIN CARDIO	LOWER BODY 3 SETS	30 MIN CARDIO	REST	15 MIN CARDIO & 1 CORE SET
7	REST	UPPER BODY 3 SETS	30 MIN CARDIO	LOWER BODY 3 SETS	30 MIN CARDIO	REST	15 MIN CARDIO & 1 CORE SET
8	REST	UPPER BODY 3 SETS	30 MIN CARDIO	LOWER BODY 3 SETS	30 MIN CARDIO	REST	15 MIN CARDIO & 1 CORE SET
9	REST	UPPER BODY 3 SETS	30 MIN CARDIO	LOWER BODY 3 SETS	30 MIN CARDIO	REST	15 MIN CARDIO & 1 CORE SET
10	REST	UPPER BODY 3 SETS	30 MIN CARDIO	LOWER BODY 3 SETS	30 MIN CARDIO	REST	15 MIN CARDIO & 1 CORE SET
11	REST	UPPER BODY 3 SETS	30 MIN CARDIO	LOWER BODY 3 SETS	30 MIN CARDIO	REST	15 MIN CARDIO & 1 CORE SET
12	REST	UPPER BODY 3 SETS	30 MIN CARDIO	LOWER BODY 3 SETS	30 MIN CARDIO	REST	15 MIN CARDIO & 1 CORE SET

NOTES

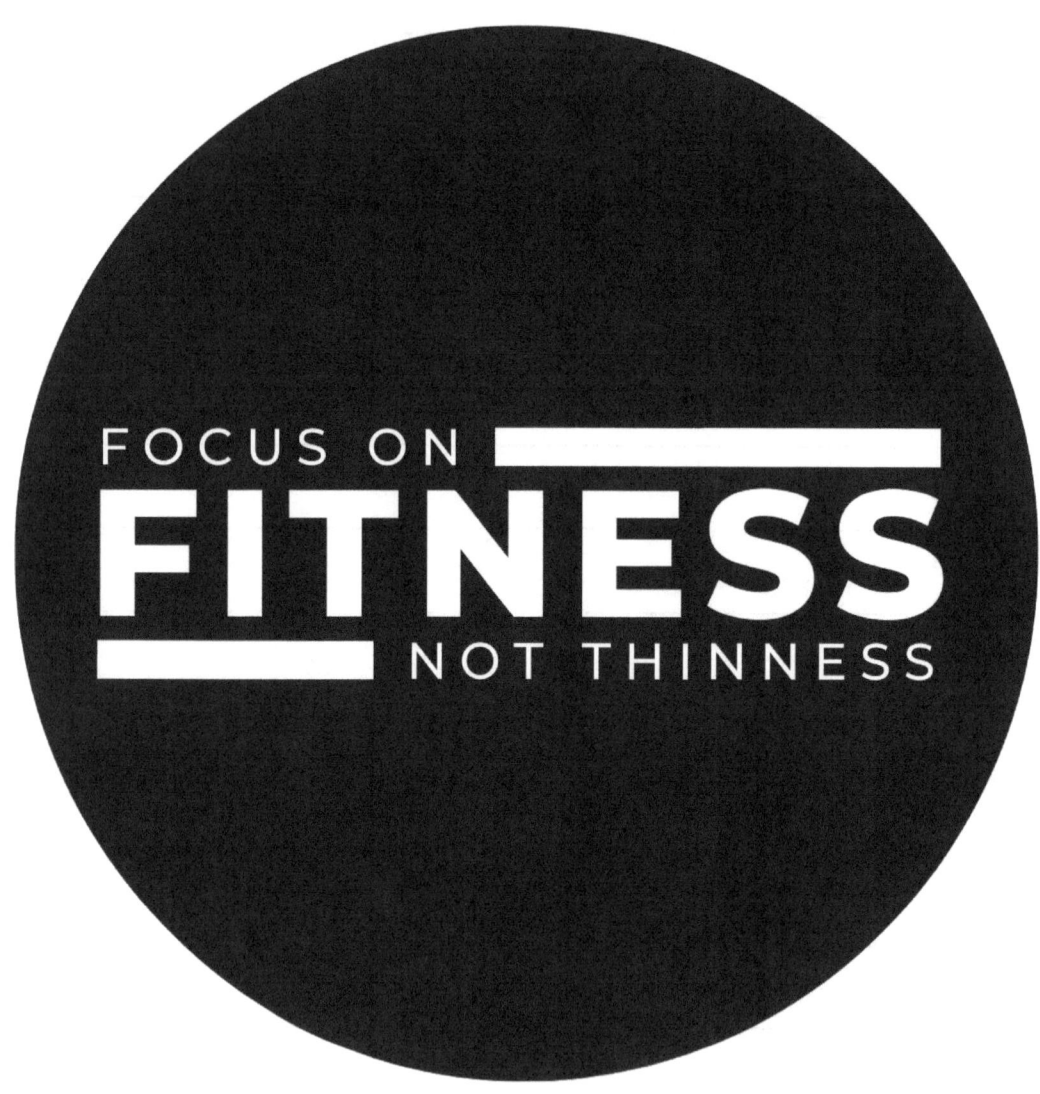

12-WEEK BLOCKS

WORKBOOK

BLOCK 1

START DATE:

END DATE:

HABIT ASSESSMENT

EAT HEALTHY WITHOUT DIETING

1. ____ I eat 2-4 cups of vegetables per day.
2. ____ I eat whole fruits rather than drinking fruit juice.
3. ____ I eat 1-3 cups of fruit per day.
4. ____ I eat a healthy breakfast everyday.
5. ____ I drink at least 8 cups of water a day (64oz).
6. ____ I eat whole wheat bread rather than white bread.
7. ____ I eat whole grain cereals rather than sugary cereals.
8. ____ I eat one or less servings of candy, cake, brownies, cookies, desserts, or similar per day.
9. ____ I eat one or less servings of potato chips, tortilla chips, crackers, or similar snacks per day.
10. ____ I eat a serving of protein with each meal.

SECTION SCORE = _____

CONTROL THOSE PORTIONS

1. ____ At each meal, I dish out a well-balanced plate.
2. ____ I only eat one serving of the meal without going back for seconds.
3. ____ When eating a dessert, unhealthy snack, or candy, I only eat one serving.
4. ____ When I eat protein in a meal (e.g. chicken, beef, fish, eggs, beans, tofu, or other proteins), it is no larger than the size of my fist.
5. ____ When I eat a starchy carbohydrate in a meal (e.g. rice, noodles, pasta, etc.), it is no larger than the size of my fist.
6. ____ When I am given a large portion of food at a restaurant, I eat half and save the other half for a later meal or share the meal with someone.
7. ____ I take my time when eating.
8. ____ I only drink water or low-fat milk with meals.
9. ____ If hungry I eat small healthy snacks in between meals.
10. ____ I avoid using excessive amounts of butter, salad dressing, or condiments.

SECTION SCORE = _____

BLOCK 1

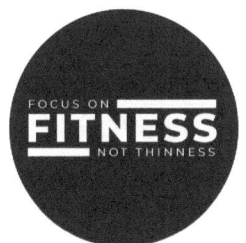

RESPONSE KEY:
0 = Never
1 = Rarely
2 = Sometimes
3 = Often
4 = Almost Always
5 = Always

HABIT ASSESSMENT

STRENGTH TRAIN

1. ____ I do strength training exercises for my arms each week.
2. ____ I do strength training exercises for my legs each week.
3. ____ I work out my core muscles each week.
4. ____ I do exercises using my body weight (e.g. pushups, squats, lunges, plank holds, etc.) as part of my strength training.
5. ____ I use weight lifting equipment (e.g. free weights or weight lifting machines) as part my strength training.
6. ____ I strength train at least two days a week.
7. ____ I give my body time to recover and rebuild by not working out the same body parts two days in a row.
8. ____ I warm up before my strength training exercises.
9. ____ I stretch after each workout to improve my flexibility.
10. ____ I refuel with protein within 30 minutes of finishing a strength training workout.

SECTION SCORE = _____

DO SOME AEROBIC EXERCISE

1. ____ I do some aerobic exercise every week.
2. ____ I take the stairs when I can, rather than the elevator.
3. ____ I park a little farther from store entrances when running errands.
4. ____ When sitting for long periods of time, I intermittently take a few minutes to get up and walk around.
5. ____ I do low-impact aerobic exercises (e.g. ride my bike, elliptical, rower, go swimming, do water aerobics, or similar).
6. ____ I do high-impact aerobic exercises (e.g. brisk walking, jogging, running, jump roping, dancing, playing basketball, soccer, tennis, or similar).
7. ____ I incorporate stretching each time I participate in aerobic exercise.
8. ____ During my aerobic exercise, the intensity is such that I could carry on a conversation rather than gasping for air.
9. ____ I do at least 150 minutes of moderate-intensity or 75 minutes of vigorous-intensity aerobic exercise each week.
10. ____ I strive to stay hydrated during and after my aerobic exercise sessions.

SECTION SCORE = _____

BLOCK 1

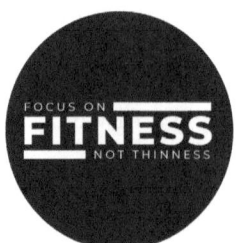

RESPONSE KEY:
0 = Never
1 = Rarely
2 = Sometimes
3 = Often
4 = Almost Always
5 = Always

ASSESSMENT RESULTS

Add up your score for each habit. The highest possible score in each category is 50; the higher the score, the better. Please refer to the chart below for interpretation.

ASSESSMENT RESULTS

EAT HEALTHY WITHOUT DIETING	
CONTROL THOSE PORTIONS	
STRENGTH TRAIN	
DO SOME AEROBIC EXERCISE	

SCORE	INTERPRETATION
41-50	EXCELLENT
31-40	GOOD
21-30	NEEDS MODERATE IMPROVEMENT
0-20	NEEDS SIGNIFICANT IMPROVEMENT

CARDIO REFERENCES

AGE	
MAXIMUM HEART RATE (220 - AGE)	
TARGET HEART RATE RANGE FOR MODERATE-INTENSITY ACTIVITY (MAX HR x 0.5 through MAX HR x 0.7)	
TARGET HEART RATE RANGE FOR VIGOROUS-INTENSITY ACTIVITY (MAX HR x 0.7 through MAX HR x 0.85)	

BODY MEASUREMENTS

DATE	
WEIGHT (lbs or kg)	
RIGHT BICEPS (inches or cm)	
WAIST (inches or cm)	
HIPS (inches or cm)	
RIGHT THIGH (inches or cm)	

BLOCK 1

MID-BLOCK MEASUREMENTS

BODY MEASUREMENTS

DATE	
WEIGHT (lbs or kg)	
RIGHT BICEPS (inches or cm)	
WAIST (inches or cm)	
HIPS (inches or cm)	
RIGHT THIGH (inches or cm)	

BLOCK 1

BLOCK 1

MEAL PLANNER

	SUN	MON	TUE	WED	THU	FRI	SAT
WEEK 1 BREAKFAST							
LUNCH							
DINNER							
WEEK 2 BREAKFAST							
LUNCH							
DINNER							
WEEK 3 BREAKFAST							
LUNCH							
DINNER							
WEEK 4 BREAKFAST							
LUNCH							
DINNER							

MEAL PLANNER

BLOCK 1

	SUN	MON	TUE	WED	THU	FRI	SAT
WEEK 5 BREAKFAST / LUNCH / DINNER							
WEEK 6 BREAKFAST / LUNCH / DINNER							
WEEK 7 BREAKFAST / LUNCH / DINNER							
WEEK 8 BREAKFAST / LUNCH / DINNER							

BLOCK 1

MEAL PLANNER

	SUN	MON	TUE	WED	THU	FRI	SAT
WEEK 9 BREAKFAST / LUNCH / DINNER							
WEEK 10 BREAKFAST / LUNCH / DINNER							
WEEK 11 BREAKFAST / LUNCH / DINNER							
WEEK 12 BREAKFAST / LUNCH / DINNER							

BLOCK 1

MY WORKOUT PLAN
12-WEEK CUSTOM WORKOUT SCHEDULE

	SUN	MON	TUE	WED	THU	FRI	SAT
1							
2							
3							
4							
5							
6							
7							
8							
9							
10							
11							
12							

BLOCK 1

BREAD & BUTTER WORKOUTS

UPPER BODY | LOWER BODY | CORE

UPPER BODY	LOWER BODY	CORE
One Arm Dumbbell Row	Squats	Crunches
Chest Press	Lunges	Leg Raises
Shoulder Press	Dead Lifts	Windshield Wipers
Biceps Curls	Leg Lifts	Mason Twists
Triceps Extensions	Calf Raises	

- Each column is a separate workout. You will only exercise one body section per scheduled workout day.

UPPER BODY WORKOUT TRACKER

BLOCK 1

	WEEK 1	WEEK 2	WEEK 3	WEEK 4	WEEK 5	WEEK 6
ONE ARM ROW	SETS- REPS- WEIGHT-	SETS- REPS- WEIGHT-	SETS- REPS- WEIGHT-	SETS- REPS- WEIGHT-	SETS- REPS- WEIGHT-	SETS- REPS- WEIGHT-
CHEST PRESS	SETS- REPS- WEIGHT-	SETS- REPS- WEIGHT-	SETS- REPS- WEIGHT-	SETS- REPS- WEIGHT-	SETS- REPS- WEIGHT-	SETS- REPS- WEIGHT-
SHOULDER PRESS	SETS- REPS- WEIGHT-	SETS- REPS- WEIGHT-	SETS- REPS- WEIGHT-	SETS- REPS- WEIGHT-	SETS- REPS- WEIGHT-	SETS- REPS- WEIGHT-
BICEPS CURLS	SETS- REPS- WEIGHT-	SETS- REPS- WEIGHT-	SETS- REPS- WEIGHT-	SETS- REPS- WEIGHT-	SETS- REPS- WEIGHT-	SETS- REPS- WEIGHT-
TRICEPS EXTENSIONS	SETS- REPS- WEIGHT-	SETS- REPS- WEIGHT-	SETS- REPS- WEIGHT-	SETS- REPS- WEIGHT-	SETS- REPS- WEIGHT-	SETS- REPS- WEIGHT-

	WEEK 7	WEEK 8	WEEK 9	WEEK 10	WEEK 11	WEEK 12
ONE ARM ROW	SETS- REPS- WEIGHT-	SETS- REPS- WEIGHT-	SETS- REPS- WEIGHT-	SETS- REPS- WEIGHT-	SETS- REPS- WEIGHT-	SETS- REPS- WEIGHT-
CHEST PRESS	SETS- REPS- WEIGHT-	SETS- REPS- WEIGHT-	SETS- REPS- WEIGHT-	SETS- REPS- WEIGHT-	SETS- REPS- WEIGHT-	SETS- REPS- WEIGHT-
SHOULDER PRESS	SETS- REPS- WEIGHT-	SETS- REPS- WEIGHT-	SETS- REPS- WEIGHT-	SETS- REPS- WEIGHT-	SETS- REPS- WEIGHT-	SETS- REPS- WEIGHT-
BICEPS CURLS	SETS- REPS- WEIGHT-	SETS- REPS- WEIGHT-	SETS- REPS- WEIGHT-	SETS- REPS- WEIGHT-	SETS- REPS- WEIGHT-	SETS- REPS- WEIGHT-
TRICEPS EXTENSIONS	SETS- REPS- WEIGHT-	SETS- REPS- WEIGHT-	SETS- REPS- WEIGHT-	SETS- REPS- WEIGHT-	SETS- REPS- WEIGHT-	SETS- REPS- WEIGHT-

BLOCK 1

LOWER BODY WORKOUT TRACKER

	WEEK 1	WEEK 2	WEEK 3	WEEK 4	WEEK 5	WEEK 6
SQUATS	SETS- REPS- WEIGHT-	SETS- REPS- WEIGHT-	SETS- REPS- WEIGHT-	SETS- REPS- WEIGHT-	SETS- REPS- WEIGHT-	SETS- REPS- WEIGHT-
LUNGES	SETS- REPS- WEIGHT-	SETS- REPS- WEIGHT-	SETS- REPS- WEIGHT-	SETS- REPS- WEIGHT-	SETS- REPS- WEIGHT-	SETS- REPS- WEIGHT-
DEAD LIFTS	SETS- REPS- WEIGHT-	SETS- REPS- WEIGHT-	SETS- REPS- WEIGHT-	SETS- REPS- WEIGHT-	SETS- REPS- WEIGHT-	SETS- REPS- WEIGHT-
LEG LIFTS	SETS- REPS- WEIGHT-	SETS- REPS- WEIGHT-	SETS- REPS- WEIGHT-	SETS- REPS- WEIGHT-	SETS- REPS- WEIGHT-	SETS- REPS- WEIGHT-
CALF RAISES	SETS- REPS- WEIGHT-	SETS- REPS- WEIGHT-	SETS- REPS- WEIGHT-	SETS- REPS- WEIGHT-	SETS- REPS- WEIGHT-	SETS- REPS- WEIGHT-

	WEEK 7	WEEK 8	WEEK 9	WEEK 10	WEEK 11	WEEK 12
SQUATS	SETS- REPS- WEIGHT-	SETS- REPS- WEIGHT-	SETS- REPS- WEIGHT-	SETS- REPS- WEIGHT-	SETS- REPS- WEIGHT-	SETS- REPS- WEIGHT-
LUNGES	SETS- REPS- WEIGHT-	SETS- REPS- WEIGHT-	SETS- REPS- WEIGHT-	SETS- REPS- WEIGHT-	SETS- REPS- WEIGHT-	SETS- REPS- WEIGHT-
DEAD LIFTS	SETS- REPS- WEIGHT-	SETS- REPS- WEIGHT-	SETS- REPS- WEIGHT-	SETS- REPS- WEIGHT-	SETS- REPS- WEIGHT-	SETS- REPS- WEIGHT-
LEG LIFTS	SETS- REPS- WEIGHT-	SETS- REPS- WEIGHT-	SETS- REPS- WEIGHT-	SETS- REPS- WEIGHT-	SETS- REPS- WEIGHT-	SETS- REPS- WEIGHT-
CALF RAISES	SETS- REPS- WEIGHT-	SETS- REPS- WEIGHT-	SETS- REPS- WEIGHT-	SETS- REPS- WEIGHT-	SETS- REPS- WEIGHT-	SETS- REPS- WEIGHT-

CORE WORKOUT TRACKER

BLOCK 1

	WEEK 1	WEEK 2	WEEK 3	WEEK 4	WEEK 5	WEEK 6
CRUNCHES	SETS- REPS- WEIGHT-	SETS- REPS- WEIGHT-	SETS- REPS- WEIGHT-	SETS- REPS- WEIGHT-	SETS- REPS- WEIGHT-	SETS- REPS- WEIGHT-
LEG RAISES	SETS- REPS- WEIGHT-	SETS- REPS- WEIGHT-	SETS- REPS- WEIGHT-	SETS- REPS- WEIGHT-	SETS- REPS- WEIGHT-	SETS- REPS- WEIGHT-
WINDSHIELD WIPERS	SETS- REPS- WEIGHT-	SETS- REPS- WEIGHT-	SETS- REPS- WEIGHT-	SETS- REPS- WEIGHT-	SETS- REPS- WEIGHT-	SETS- REPS- WEIGHT-
MASON TWISTS	SETS- REPS- WEIGHT-	SETS- REPS- WEIGHT-	SETS- REPS- WEIGHT-	SETS- REPS- WEIGHT-	SETS- REPS- WEIGHT-	SETS- REPS- WEIGHT-

	WEEK 7	WEEK 8	WEEK 9	WEEK 10	WEEK 11	WEEK 12
CRUNCHES	SETS- REPS- WEIGHT-	SETS- REPS- WEIGHT-	SETS- REPS- WEIGHT-	SETS- REPS- WEIGHT-	SETS- REPS- WEIGHT-	SETS- REPS- WEIGHT-
LEG RAISES	SETS- REPS- WEIGHT-	SETS- REPS- WEIGHT-	SETS- REPS- WEIGHT-	SETS- REPS- WEIGHT-	SETS- REPS- WEIGHT-	SETS- REPS- WEIGHT-
WINDSHIELD WIPERS	SETS- REPS- WEIGHT-	SETS- REPS- WEIGHT-	SETS- REPS- WEIGHT-	SETS- REPS- WEIGHT-	SETS- REPS- WEIGHT-	SETS- REPS- WEIGHT-
MASON TWISTS	SETS- REPS- WEIGHT-	SETS- REPS- WEIGHT-	SETS- REPS- WEIGHT-	SETS- REPS- WEIGHT-	SETS- REPS- WEIGHT-	SETS- REPS- WEIGHT-

NOTES

NOTES

BLOCK 2

START DATE:

END DATE:

HABIT ASSESSMENT

EAT HEALTHY WITHOUT DIETING

1. ____ I eat 2-4 cups of vegetables per day.
2. ____ I eat whole fruits rather than drinking fruit juice.
3. ____ I eat 1-3 cups of fruit per day.
4. ____ I eat a healthy breakfast everyday.
5. ____ I drink at least 8 cups of water a day (64oz).
6. ____ I eat whole wheat bread rather than white bread.
7. ____ I eat whole grain cereals rather than sugary cereals.
8. ____ I eat one or less servings of candy, cake, brownies, cookies, desserts, or similar per day.
9. ____ I eat one or less servings of potato chips, tortilla chips, crackers, or similar snacks per day.
10. ____ I eat a serving of protein with each meal.

SECTION SCORE = _____

CONTROL THOSE PORTIONS

1. ____ At each meal, I dish out a well-balanced plate.
2. ____ I only eat one serving of the meal without going back for seconds.
3. ____ When eating a dessert, unhealthy snack, or candy, I only eat one serving.
4. ____ When I eat protein in a meal (e.g. chicken, beef, fish, eggs, beans, tofu, or other proteins), it is no larger than the size of my fist.
5. ____ When I eat a starchy carbohydrate in a meal (e.g. rice, noodles, pasta, etc.), it is no larger than the size of my fist.
6. ____ When I am given a large portion of food at a restaurant, I eat half and save the other half for a later meal or share the meal with someone.
7. ____ I take my time when eating.
8. ____ I only drink water or low-fat milk with meals.
9. ____ If hungry I eat small healthy snacks in between meals.
10. ____ I avoid using excessive amounts of butter, salad dressing, or condiments.

SECTION SCORE = _____

BLOCK 2

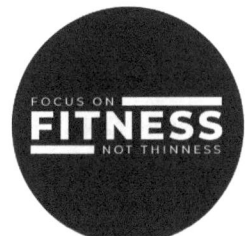

RESPONSE KEY:
0 = Never
1 = Rarely
2 = Sometimes
3 = Often
4 = Almost Always
5 = Always

HABIT ASSESSMENT

STRENGTH TRAIN

1. ____ I do strength training exercises for my arms each week.
2. ____ I do strength training exercises for my legs each week.
3. ____ I work out my core muscles each week.
4. ____ I do exercises using my body weight (e.g. pushups, squats, lunges, plank holds, etc.) as part of my strength training.
5. ____ I use weight lifting equipment (e.g. free weights or weight lifting machines) as part my strength training.
6. ____ I strength train at least two days a week.
7. ____ I give my body time to recover and rebuild by not working out the same body parts two days in a row.
8. ____ I warm up before my strength training exercises.
9. ____ I stretch after each workout to improve my flexibility.
10. ____ I refuel with protein within 30 minutes of finishing a strength training workout.

SECTION SCORE = _____

DO SOME AEROBIC EXERCISE

1. ____ I do some aerobic exercise every week.
2. ____ I take the stairs when I can, rather than the elevator.
3. ____ I park a little farther from store entrances when running errands.
4. ____ When sitting for long periods of time, I intermittently take a few minutes to get up and walk around.
5. ____ I do low-impact aerobic exercises (e.g. ride my bike, elliptical, rower, go swimming, do water aerobics, or similar).
6. ____ I do high-impact aerobic exercises (e.g. brisk walking, jogging, running, jump roping, dancing, playing basketball, soccer, tennis, or similar).
7. ____ I incorporate stretching each time I participate in aerobic exercise.
8. ____ During my aerobic exercise, the intensity is such that I could carry on a conversation rather than gasping for air.
9. ____ I do at least 150 minutes of moderate-intensity or 75 minutes of vigorous-intensity aerobic exercise each week.
10. ____ I strive to stay hydrated during and after my aerobic exercise sessions.

SECTION SCORE = _____

BLOCK 2

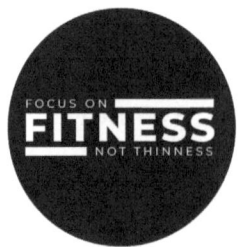

RESPONSE KEY:
0 = Never
1 = Rarely
2 = Sometimes
3 = Often
4 = Almost Always
5 = Always

ASSESSMENT RESULTS

Add up your score for each habit. The highest possible score in each category is 50; the higher the score, the better. Please refer to the chart below for interpretation.

ASSESSMENT RESULTS

EAT HEALTHY WITHOUT DIETING	
CONTROL THOSE PORTIONS	
STRENGTH TRAIN	
DO SOME AEROBIC EXERCISE	

SCORE	INTERPRETATION
41-50	EXCELLENT
31-40	GOOD
21-30	NEEDS MODERATE IMPROVEMENT
0-20	NEEDS SIGNIFICANT IMPROVEMENT

CARDIO REFERENCES

AGE	
MAXIMUM HEART RATE (220 - AGE)	
TARGET HEART RATE RANGE FOR MODERATE-INTENSITY ACTIVITY (MAX HR x 0.5 through MAX HR x 0.7)	
TARGET HEART RATE RANGE FOR VIGOROUS-INTENSITY ACTIVITY (MAX HR x 0.7 through MAX HR x 0.85)	

BODY MEASUREMENTS

DATE	
WEIGHT (lbs or kg)	
RIGHT BICEPS (inches or cm)	
WAIST (inches or cm)	
HIPS (inches or cm)	
RIGHT THIGH (inches or cm)	

MID-BLOCK MEASUREMENTS

BODY MEASUREMENTS

DATE	
WEIGHT (lbs or kg)	
RIGHT BICEPS (inches or cm)	
WAIST (inches or cm)	
HIPS (inches or cm)	
RIGHT THIGH (inches or cm)	

BLOCK 2

BLOCK 2

MEAL PLANNER

	SUN	MON	TUE	WED	THU	FRI	SAT
WEEK 1 BREAKFAST / LUNCH / DINNER							
WEEK 2 BREAKFAST / LUNCH / DINNER							
WEEK 3 BREAKFAST / LUNCH / DINNER							
WEEK 4 BREAKFAST / LUNCH / DINNER							

MEAL PLANNER

BLOCK 2

	SUN	MON	TUE	WED	THU	FRI	SAT
WEEK 5 BREAKFAST / LUNCH / DINNER							
WEEK 6 BREAKFAST / LUNCH / DINNER							
WEEK 7 BREAKFAST / LUNCH / DINNER							
WEEK 8 BREAKFAST / LUNCH / DINNER							

BLOCK 2

MEAL PLANNER

	SUN	MON	TUE	WED	THU	FRI	SAT
WEEK 9 BREAKFAST							
LUNCH							
DINNER							
WEEK 10 BREAKFAST							
LUNCH							
DINNER							
WEEK 11 BREAKFAST							
LUNCH							
DINNER							
WEEK 12 BREAKFAST							
LUNCH							
DINNER							

MY WORKOUT PLAN

12-WEEK CUSTOM WORKOUT SCHEDULE

BLOCK 2

	SUN	MON	TUE	WED	THU	FRI	SAT
1							
2							
3							
4							
5							
6							
7							
8							
9							
10							
11							
12							

BLOCK 2

BREAD & BUTTER WORKOUTS

UPPER BODY **LOWER BODY** **CORE**

Upper Body	Lower Body	Core
One Arm Dumbbell Row	Squats	Crunches
Chest Press	Lunges	Leg Raises
Shoulder Press	Dead Lifts	Windshield Wipers
Biceps Curls	Leg Lifts	Mason Twists
Triceps Extensions	Calf Raises	

- Each column is a separate workout. You will only exercise one body section per scheduled workout day.

BLOCK 2

UPPER BODY WORKOUT TRACKER

	WEEK 1	WEEK 2	WEEK 3	WEEK 4	WEEK 5	WEEK 6
ONE ARM ROW	SETS- REPS- WEIGHT-	SETS- REPS- WEIGHT-	SETS- REPS- WEIGHT-	SETS- REPS- WEIGHT-	SETS- REPS- WEIGHT-	SETS- REPS- WEIGHT-
CHEST PRESS	SETS- REPS- WEIGHT-	SETS- REPS- WEIGHT-	SETS- REPS- WEIGHT-	SETS- REPS- WEIGHT-	SETS- REPS- WEIGHT-	SETS- REPS- WEIGHT-
SHOULDER PRESS	SETS- REPS- WEIGHT-	SETS- REPS- WEIGHT-	SETS- REPS- WEIGHT-	SETS- REPS- WEIGHT-	SETS- REPS- WEIGHT-	SETS- REPS- WEIGHT-
BICEPS CURLS	SETS- REPS- WEIGHT-	SETS- REPS- WEIGHT-	SETS- REPS- WEIGHT-	SETS- REPS- WEIGHT-	SETS- REPS- WEIGHT-	SETS- REPS- WEIGHT-
TRICEPS EXTENSIONS	SETS- REPS- WEIGHT-	SETS- REPS- WEIGHT-	SETS- REPS- WEIGHT-	SETS- REPS- WEIGHT-	SETS- REPS- WEIGHT-	SETS- REPS- WEIGHT-

	WEEK 7	WEEK 8	WEEK 9	WEEK 10	WEEK 11	WEEK 12
ONE ARM ROW	SETS- REPS- WEIGHT-	SETS- REPS- WEIGHT-	SETS- REPS- WEIGHT-	SETS- REPS- WEIGHT-	SETS- REPS- WEIGHT-	SETS- REPS- WEIGHT-
CHEST PRESS	SETS- REPS- WEIGHT-	SETS- REPS- WEIGHT-	SETS- REPS- WEIGHT-	SETS- REPS- WEIGHT-	SETS- REPS- WEIGHT-	SETS- REPS- WEIGHT-
SHOULDER PRESS	SETS- REPS- WEIGHT-	SETS- REPS- WEIGHT-	SETS- REPS- WEIGHT-	SETS- REPS- WEIGHT-	SETS- REPS- WEIGHT-	SETS- REPS- WEIGHT-
BICEPS CURLS	SETS- REPS- WEIGHT-	SETS- REPS- WEIGHT-	SETS- REPS- WEIGHT-	SETS- REPS- WEIGHT-	SETS- REPS- WEIGHT-	SETS- REPS- WEIGHT-
TRICEPS EXTENSIONS	SETS- REPS- WEIGHT-	SETS- REPS- WEIGHT-	SETS- REPS- WEIGHT-	SETS- REPS- WEIGHT-	SETS- REPS- WEIGHT-	SETS- REPS- WEIGHT-

BLOCK 2

LOWER BODY WORKOUT TRACKER

	WEEK 1	WEEK 2	WEEK 3	WEEK 4	WEEK 5	WEEK 6
SQUATS	SETS- REPS- WEIGHT-	SETS- REPS- WEIGHT-	SETS- REPS- WEIGHT-	SETS- REPS- WEIGHT-	SETS- REPS- WEIGHT-	SETS- REPS- WEIGHT-
LUNGES	SETS- REPS- WEIGHT-	SETS- REPS- WEIGHT-	SETS- REPS- WEIGHT-	SETS- REPS- WEIGHT-	SETS- REPS- WEIGHT-	SETS- REPS- WEIGHT-
DEAD LIFTS	SETS- REPS- WEIGHT-	SETS- REPS- WEIGHT-	SETS- REPS- WEIGHT-	SETS- REPS- WEIGHT-	SETS- REPS- WEIGHT-	SETS- REPS- WEIGHT-
LEG LIFTS	SETS- REPS- WEIGHT-	SETS- REPS- WEIGHT-	SETS- REPS- WEIGHT-	SETS- REPS- WEIGHT-	SETS- REPS- WEIGHT-	SETS- REPS- WEIGHT-
CALF RAISES	SETS- REPS- WEIGHT-	SETS- REPS- WEIGHT-	SETS- REPS- WEIGHT-	SETS- REPS- WEIGHT-	SETS- REPS- WEIGHT-	SETS- REPS- WEIGHT-

	WEEK 7	WEEK 8	WEEK 9	WEEK 10	WEEK 11	WEEK 12
SQUATS	SETS- REPS- WEIGHT-	SETS- REPS- WEIGHT-	SETS- REPS- WEIGHT-	SETS- REPS- WEIGHT-	SETS- REPS- WEIGHT-	SETS- REPS- WEIGHT-
LUNGES	SETS- REPS- WEIGHT-	SETS- REPS- WEIGHT-	SETS- REPS- WEIGHT-	SETS- REPS- WEIGHT-	SETS- REPS- WEIGHT-	SETS- REPS- WEIGHT-
DEAD LIFTS	SETS- REPS- WEIGHT-	SETS- REPS- WEIGHT-	SETS- REPS- WEIGHT-	SETS- REPS- WEIGHT-	SETS- REPS- WEIGHT-	SETS- REPS- WEIGHT-
LEG LIFTS	SETS- REPS- WEIGHT-	SETS- REPS- WEIGHT-	SETS- REPS- WEIGHT-	SETS- REPS- WEIGHT-	SETS- REPS- WEIGHT-	SETS- REPS- WEIGHT-
CALF RAISES	SETS- REPS- WEIGHT-	SETS- REPS- WEIGHT-	SETS- REPS- WEIGHT-	SETS- REPS- WEIGHT-	SETS- REPS- WEIGHT-	SETS- REPS- WEIGHT-

CORE WORKOUT TRACKER

BLOCK 2

	WEEK 1	WEEK 2	WEEK 3	WEEK 4	WEEK 5	WEEK 6
CRUNCHES	SETS- REPS- WEIGHT-	SETS- REPS- WEIGHT-	SETS- REPS- WEIGHT-	SETS- REPS- WEIGHT-	SETS- REPS- WEIGHT-	SETS- REPS- WEIGHT-
LEG RAISES	SETS- REPS- WEIGHT-	SETS- REPS- WEIGHT-	SETS- REPS- WEIGHT-	SETS- REPS- WEIGHT-	SETS- REPS- WEIGHT-	SETS- REPS- WEIGHT-
WINDSHIELD WIPERS	SETS- REPS- WEIGHT-	SETS- REPS- WEIGHT-	SETS- REPS- WEIGHT-	SETS- REPS- WEIGHT-	SETS- REPS- WEIGHT-	SETS- REPS- WEIGHT-
MASON TWISTS	SETS- REPS- WEIGHT-	SETS- REPS- WEIGHT-	SETS- REPS- WEIGHT-	SETS- REPS- WEIGHT-	SETS- REPS- WEIGHT-	SETS- REPS- WEIGHT-

	WEEK 7	WEEK 8	WEEK 9	WEEK 10	WEEK 11	WEEK 12
CRUNCHES	SETS- REPS- WEIGHT-	SETS- REPS- WEIGHT-	SETS- REPS- WEIGHT-	SETS- REPS- WEIGHT-	SETS- REPS- WEIGHT-	SETS- REPS- WEIGHT-
LEG RAISES	SETS- REPS- WEIGHT-	SETS- REPS- WEIGHT-	SETS- REPS- WEIGHT-	SETS- REPS- WEIGHT-	SETS- REPS- WEIGHT-	SETS- REPS- WEIGHT-
WINDSHIELD WIPERS	SETS- REPS- WEIGHT-	SETS- REPS- WEIGHT-	SETS- REPS- WEIGHT-	SETS- REPS- WEIGHT-	SETS- REPS- WEIGHT-	SETS- REPS- WEIGHT-
MASON TWISTS	SETS- REPS- WEIGHT-	SETS- REPS- WEIGHT-	SETS- REPS- WEIGHT-	SETS- REPS- WEIGHT-	SETS- REPS- WEIGHT-	SETS- REPS- WEIGHT-

NOTES

NOTES

BLOCK 3

START DATE:

END DATE:

HABIT ASSESSMENT

EAT HEALTHY WITHOUT DIETING

1. ____ I eat 2-4 cups of vegetables per day.
2. ____ I eat whole fruits rather than drinking fruit juice.
3. ____ I eat 1-3 cups of fruit per day.
4. ____ I eat a healthy breakfast everyday.
5. ____ I drink at least 8 cups of water a day (64oz).
6. ____ I eat whole wheat bread rather than white bread.
7. ____ I eat whole grain cereals rather than sugary cereals.
8. ____ I eat one or less servings of candy, cake, brownies, cookies, desserts, or similar per day.
9. ____ I eat one or less servings of potato chips, tortilla chips, crackers, or similar snacks per day.
10. ____ I eat a serving of protein with each meal.

SECTION SCORE = _____

CONTROL THOSE PORTIONS

1. ____ At each meal, I dish out a well-balanced plate.
2. ____ I only eat one serving of the meal without going back for seconds.
3. ____ When eating a dessert, unhealthy snack, or candy, I only eat one serving.
4. ____ When I eat protein in a meal (e.g. chicken, beef, fish, eggs, beans, tofu, or other proteins), it is no larger than the size of my fist.
5. ____ When I eat a starchy carbohydrate in a meal (e.g. rice, noodles, pasta, etc.), it is no larger than the size of my fist.
6. ____ When I am given a large portion of food at a restaurant, I eat half and save the other half for a later meal or share the meal with someone.
7. ____ I take my time when eating.
8. ____ I only drink water or low-fat milk with meals.
9. ____ If hungry I eat small healthy snacks in between meals.
10. ____ I avoid using excessive amounts of butter, salad dressing, or condiments.

SECTION SCORE = _____

BLOCK 3

RESPONSE KEY:
0 = Never
1 = Rarely
2 = Sometimes
3 = Often
4 = Almost Always
5 = Always

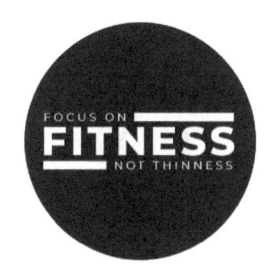

HABIT ASSESSMENT

STRENGTH TRAIN

1. ____ I do strength training exercises for my arms each week.
2. ____ I do strength training exercises for my legs each week.
3. ____ I work out my core muscles each week.
4. ____ I do exercises using my body weight (e.g. pushups, squats, lunges, plank holds, etc.) as part of my strength training.
5. ____ I use weight lifting equipment (e.g. free weights or weight lifting machines) as part my strength training.
6. ____ I strength train at least two days a week.
7. ____ I give my body time to recover and rebuild by not working out the same body parts two days in a row.
8. ____ I warm up before my strength training exercises.
9. ____ I stretch after each workout to improve my flexibility.
10. ____ I refuel with protein within 30 minutes of finishing a strength training workout.

SECTION SCORE = _____

DO SOME AEROBIC EXERCISE

1. ____ I do some aerobic exercise every week.
2. ____ I take the stairs when I can, rather than the elevator.
3. ____ I park a little farther from store entrances when running errands.
4. ____ When sitting for long periods of time, I intermittently take a few minutes to get up and walk around.
5. ____ I do low-impact aerobic exercises (e.g. ride my bike, elliptical, rower, go swimming, do water aerobics, or similar).
6. ____ I do high-impact aerobic exercises (e.g. brisk walking, jogging, running, jump roping, dancing, playing basketball, soccer, tennis, or similar).
7. ____ I incorporate stretching each time I participate in aerobic exercise.
8. ____ During my aerobic exercise, the intensity is such that I could carry on a conversation rather than gasping for air.
9. ____ I do at least 150 minutes of moderate-intensity or 75 minutes of vigorous-intensity aerobic exercise each week.
10. ____ I strive to stay hydrated during and after my aerobic exercise sessions.

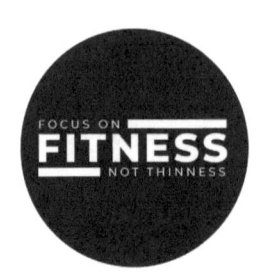

SECTION SCORE = _____

BLOCK 3

RESPONSE KEY:
0 = Never
1 = Rarely
2 = Sometimes
3 = Often
4 = Almost Always
5 = Always

ASSESSMENT RESULTS

Add up your score for each habit. The highest possible score in each category is 50; the higher the score, the better. Please refer to the chart below for interpretation.

ASSESSMENT RESULTS

EAT HEALTHY WITHOUT DIETING	
CONTROL THOSE PORTIONS	
STRENGTH TRAIN	
DO SOME AEROBIC EXERCISE	

SCORE	INTERPRETATION
41-50	EXCELLENT
31-40	GOOD
21-30	NEEDS MODERATE IMPROVEMENT
0-20	NEEDS SIGNIFICANT IMPROVEMENT

BLOCK 3

CARDIO REFERENCES

AGE	
MAXIMUM HEART RATE (220 - AGE)	
TARGET HEART RATE RANGE FOR MODERATE-INTENSITY ACTIVITY (MAX HR x 0.5 through MAX HR x 0.7)	
TARGET HEART RATE RANGE FOR VIGOROUS-INTENSITY ACTIVITY (MAX HR x 0.7 through MAX HR x 0.85)	

BODY MEASUREMENTS

DATE	
WEIGHT (lbs or kg)	
RIGHT BICEPS (inches or cm)	
WAIST (inches or cm)	
HIPS (inches or cm)	
RIGHT THIGH (inches or cm)	

BLOCK 3

MID-BLOCK MEASUREMENTS

BODY MEASUREMENTS

DATE	
WEIGHT (lbs or kg)	
RIGHT BICEPS (inches or cm)	
WAIST (inches or cm)	
HIPS (inches or cm)	
RIGHT THIGH (inches or cm)	

BLOCK 3

BLOCK 3

MEAL PLANNER

	SUN	MON	TUE	WED	THU	FRI	SAT
WEEK 1 BREAKFAST							
LUNCH							
DINNER							
WEEK 2 BREAKFAST							
LUNCH							
DINNER							
WEEK 3 BREAKFAST							
LUNCH							
DINNER							
WEEK 4 BREAKFAST							
LUNCH							
DINNER							

MEAL PLANNER

BLOCK 3

	SUN	MON	TUE	WED	THU	FRI	SAT
WEEK 5 BREAKFAST							
LUNCH							
DINNER							
WEEK 6 BREAKFAST							
LUNCH							
DINNER							
WEEK 7 BREAKFAST							
LUNCH							
DINNER							
WEEK 8 BREAKFAST							
LUNCH							
DINNER							

BLOCK 3

MEAL PLANNER

	SUN	MON	TUE	WED	THU	FRI	SAT
WEEK 9 BREAKFAST							
LUNCH							
DINNER							
WEEK 10 BREAKFAST							
LUNCH							
DINNER							
WEEK 11 BREAKFAST							
LUNCH							
DINNER							
WEEK 12 BREAKFAST							
LUNCH							
DINNER							

MY WORKOUT PLAN

12-WEEK CUSTOM WORKOUT SCHEDULE

BLOCK 3

	SUN	MON	TUE	WED	THU	FRI	SAT
1							
2							
3							
4							
5							
6							
7							
8							
9							
10							
11							
12							

BLOCK 3

BREAD & BUTTER WORKOUTS

UPPER BODY	LOWER BODY	CORE
One Arm Dumbbell Row	Squats	Crunches
Chest Press	Lunges	Leg Raises
Shoulder Press	Dead Lifts	Windshield Wipers
Biceps Curls	Leg Lifts	Mason Twists
Triceps Extensions	Calf Raises	

- Each column is a separate workout. You will only exercise one body section per scheduled workout day.

UPPER BODY WORKOUT TRACKER

BLOCK 3

	WEEK 1	WEEK 2	WEEK 3	WEEK 4	WEEK 5	WEEK 6
ONE ARM ROW	SETS- REPS- WEIGHT-	SETS- REPS- WEIGHT-	SETS- REPS- WEIGHT-	SETS- REPS- WEIGHT-	SETS- REPS- WEIGHT-	SETS- REPS- WEIGHT-
CHEST PRESS	SETS- REPS- WEIGHT-	SETS- REPS- WEIGHT-	SETS- REPS- WEIGHT-	SETS- REPS- WEIGHT-	SETS- REPS- WEIGHT-	SETS- REPS- WEIGHT-
SHOULDER PRESS	SETS- REPS- WEIGHT-	SETS- REPS- WEIGHT-	SETS- REPS- WEIGHT-	SETS- REPS- WEIGHT-	SETS- REPS- WEIGHT-	SETS- REPS- WEIGHT-
BICEPS CURLS	SETS- REPS- WEIGHT-	SETS- REPS- WEIGHT-	SETS- REPS- WEIGHT-	SETS- REPS- WEIGHT-	SETS- REPS- WEIGHT-	SETS- REPS- WEIGHT-
TRICEPS EXTENSIONS	SETS- REPS- WEIGHT-	SETS- REPS- WEIGHT-	SETS- REPS- WEIGHT-	SETS- REPS- WEIGHT-	SETS- REPS- WEIGHT-	SETS- REPS- WEIGHT-

	WEEK 7	WEEK 8	WEEK 9	WEEK 10	WEEK 11	WEEK 12
ONE ARM ROW	SETS- REPS- WEIGHT-	SETS- REPS- WEIGHT-	SETS- REPS- WEIGHT-	SETS- REPS- WEIGHT-	SETS- REPS- WEIGHT-	SETS- REPS- WEIGHT-
CHEST PRESS	SETS- REPS- WEIGHT-	SETS- REPS- WEIGHT-	SETS- REPS- WEIGHT-	SETS- REPS- WEIGHT-	SETS- REPS- WEIGHT-	SETS- REPS- WEIGHT-
SHOULDER PRESS	SETS- REPS- WEIGHT-	SETS- REPS- WEIGHT-	SETS- REPS- WEIGHT-	SETS- REPS- WEIGHT-	SETS- REPS- WEIGHT-	SETS- REPS- WEIGHT-
BICEPS CURLS	SETS- REPS- WEIGHT-	SETS- REPS- WEIGHT-	SETS- REPS- WEIGHT-	SETS- REPS- WEIGHT-	SETS- REPS- WEIGHT-	SETS- REPS- WEIGHT-
TRICEPS EXTENSIONS	SETS- REPS- WEIGHT-	SETS- REPS- WEIGHT-	SETS- REPS- WEIGHT-	SETS- REPS- WEIGHT-	SETS- REPS- WEIGHT-	SETS- REPS- WEIGHT-

BLOCK 3

LOWER BODY WORKOUT TRACKER

	WEEK 1	WEEK 2	WEEK 3	WEEK 4	WEEK 5	WEEK 6
SQUATS	SETS- REPS- WEIGHT-	SETS- REPS- WEIGHT-	SETS- REPS- WEIGHT-	SETS- REPS- WEIGHT-	SETS- REPS- WEIGHT-	SETS- REPS- WEIGHT-
LUNGES	SETS- REPS- WEIGHT-	SETS- REPS- WEIGHT-	SETS- REPS- WEIGHT-	SETS- REPS- WEIGHT-	SETS- REPS- WEIGHT-	SETS- REPS- WEIGHT-
DEAD LIFTS	SETS- REPS- WEIGHT-	SETS- REPS- WEIGHT-	SETS- REPS- WEIGHT-	SETS- REPS- WEIGHT-	SETS- REPS- WEIGHT-	SETS- REPS- WEIGHT-
LEG LIFTS	SETS- REPS- WEIGHT-	SETS- REPS- WEIGHT-	SETS- REPS- WEIGHT-	SETS- REPS- WEIGHT-	SETS- REPS- WEIGHT-	SETS- REPS- WEIGHT-
CALF RAISES	SETS- REPS- WEIGHT-	SETS- REPS- WEIGHT-	SETS- REPS- WEIGHT-	SETS- REPS- WEIGHT-	SETS- REPS- WEIGHT-	SETS- REPS- WEIGHT-

	WEEK 7	WEEK 8	WEEK 9	WEEK 10	WEEK 11	WEEK 12
SQUATS	SETS- REPS- WEIGHT-	SETS- REPS- WEIGHT-	SETS- REPS- WEIGHT-	SETS- REPS- WEIGHT-	SETS- REPS- WEIGHT-	SETS- REPS- WEIGHT-
LUNGES	SETS- REPS- WEIGHT-	SETS- REPS- WEIGHT-	SETS- REPS- WEIGHT-	SETS- REPS- WEIGHT-	SETS- REPS- WEIGHT-	SETS- REPS- WEIGHT-
DEAD LIFTS	SETS- REPS- WEIGHT-	SETS- REPS- WEIGHT-	SETS- REPS- WEIGHT-	SETS- REPS- WEIGHT-	SETS- REPS- WEIGHT-	SETS- REPS- WEIGHT-
LEG LIFTS	SETS- REPS- WEIGHT-	SETS- REPS- WEIGHT-	SETS- REPS- WEIGHT-	SETS- REPS- WEIGHT-	SETS- REPS- WEIGHT-	SETS- REPS- WEIGHT-
CALF RAISES	SETS- REPS- WEIGHT-	SETS- REPS- WEIGHT-	SETS- REPS- WEIGHT-	SETS- REPS- WEIGHT-	SETS- REPS- WEIGHT-	SETS- REPS- WEIGHT-

CORE WORKOUT TRACKER

BLOCK 3

	WEEK 1	WEEK 2	WEEK 3	WEEK 4	WEEK 5	WEEK 6
CRUNCHES	SETS- REPS- WEIGHT-	SETS- REPS- WEIGHT-	SETS- REPS- WEIGHT-	SETS- REPS- WEIGHT-	SETS- REPS- WEIGHT-	SETS- REPS- WEIGHT-
LEG RAISES	SETS- REPS- WEIGHT-	SETS- REPS- WEIGHT-	SETS- REPS- WEIGHT-	SETS- REPS- WEIGHT-	SETS- REPS- WEIGHT-	SETS- REPS- WEIGHT-
WINDSHIELD WIPERS	SETS- REPS- WEIGHT-	SETS- REPS- WEIGHT-	SETS- REPS- WEIGHT-	SETS- REPS- WEIGHT-	SETS- REPS- WEIGHT-	SETS- REPS- WEIGHT-
MASON TWISTS	SETS- REPS- WEIGHT-	SETS- REPS- WEIGHT-	SETS- REPS- WEIGHT-	SETS- REPS- WEIGHT-	SETS- REPS- WEIGHT-	SETS- REPS- WEIGHT-

	WEEK 7	WEEK 8	WEEK 9	WEEK 10	WEEK 11	WEEK 12
CRUNCHES	SETS- REPS- WEIGHT-	SETS- REPS- WEIGHT-	SETS- REPS- WEIGHT-	SETS- REPS- WEIGHT-	SETS- REPS- WEIGHT-	SETS- REPS- WEIGHT-
LEG RAISES	SETS- REPS- WEIGHT-	SETS- REPS- WEIGHT-	SETS- REPS- WEIGHT-	SETS- REPS- WEIGHT-	SETS- REPS- WEIGHT-	SETS- REPS- WEIGHT-
WINDSHIELD WIPERS	SETS- REPS- WEIGHT-	SETS- REPS- WEIGHT-	SETS- REPS- WEIGHT-	SETS- REPS- WEIGHT-	SETS- REPS- WEIGHT-	SETS- REPS- WEIGHT-
MASON TWISTS	SETS- REPS- WEIGHT-	SETS- REPS- WEIGHT-	SETS- REPS- WEIGHT-	SETS- REPS- WEIGHT-	SETS- REPS- WEIGHT-	SETS- REPS- WEIGHT-

NOTES

NOTES

BLOCK 4

START DATE:

END DATE:

HABIT ASSESSMENT

EAT HEALTHY WITHOUT DIETING

1. ____ I eat 2-4 cups of vegetables per day.
2. ____ I eat whole fruits rather than drinking fruit juice.
3. ____ I eat 1-3 cups of fruit per day.
4. ____ I eat a healthy breakfast everyday.
5. ____ I drink at least 8 cups of water a day (64oz).
6. ____ I eat whole wheat bread rather than white bread.
7. ____ I eat whole grain cereals rather than sugary cereals.
8. ____ I eat one or less servings of candy, cake, brownies, cookies, desserts, or similar per day.
9. ____ I eat one or less servings of potato chips, tortilla chips, crackers, or similar snacks per day.
10. ____ I eat a serving of protein with each meal.

SECTION SCORE = _____

CONTROL THOSE PORTIONS

1. ____ At each meal, I dish out a well-balanced plate.
2. ____ I only eat one serving of the meal without going back for seconds.
3. ____ When eating a dessert, unhealthy snack, or candy, I only eat one serving.
4. ____ When I eat protein in a meal (e.g. chicken, beef, fish, eggs, beans, tofu, or other proteins), it is no larger than the size of my fist.
5. ____ When I eat a starchy carbohydrate in a meal (e.g. rice, noodles, pasta, etc.), it is no larger than the size of my fist.
6. ____ When I am given a large portion of food at a restaurant, I eat half and save the other half for a later meal or share the meal with someone.
7. ____ I take my time when eating.
8. ____ I only drink water or low-fat milk with meals.
9. ____ If hungry I eat small healthy snacks in between meals.
10. ____ I avoid using excessive amounts of butter, salad dressing, or condiments.

SECTION SCORE = _____

BLOCK 4

RESPONSE KEY:
0 = Never
1 = Rarely
2 = Sometimes
3 = Often
4 = Almost Always
5 = Always

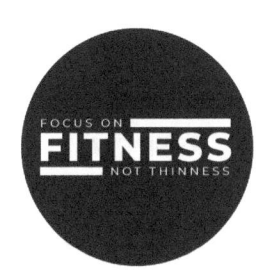

HABIT ASSESSMENT

STRENGTH TRAIN

1. ____ I do strength training exercises for my arms each week.
2. ____ I do strength training exercises for my legs each week.
3. ____ I work out my core muscles each week.
4. ____ I do exercises using my body weight (e.g. pushups, squats, lunges, plank holds, etc.) as part of my strength training.
5. ____ I use weight lifting equipment (e.g. free weights or weight lifting machines) as part my strength training.
6. ____ I strength train at least two days a week.
7. ____ I give my body time to recover and rebuild by not working out the same body parts two days in a row.
8. ____ I warm up before my strength training exercises.
9. ____ I stretch after each workout to improve my flexibility.
10. ____ I refuel with protein within 30 minutes of finishing a strength training workout.

SECTION SCORE = _____

DO SOME AEROBIC EXERCISE

1. ____ I do some aerobic exercise every week.
2. ____ I take the stairs when I can, rather than the elevator.
3. ____ I park a little farther from store entrances when running errands.
4. ____ When sitting for long periods of time, I intermittently take a few minutes to get up and walk around.
5. ____ I do low-impact aerobic exercises (e.g. ride my bike, elliptical, rower, go swimming, do water aerobics, or similar).
6. ____ I do high-impact aerobic exercises (e.g. brisk walking, jogging, running, jump roping, dancing, playing basketball, soccer, tennis, or similar).
7. ____ I incorporate stretching each time I participate in aerobic exercise.
8. ____ During my aerobic exercise, the intensity is such that I could carry on a conversation rather than gasping for air.
9. ____ I do at least 150 minutes of moderate-intensity or 75 minutes of vigorous-intensity aerobic exercise each week.
10. ____ I strive to stay hydrated during and after my aerobic exercise sessions.

SECTION SCORE = _____

BLOCK 4

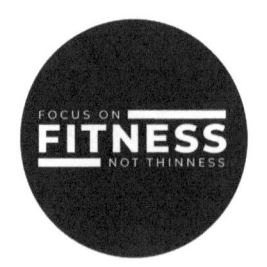

RESPONSE KEY:
0 = Never
1 = Rarely
2 = Sometimes
3 = Often
4 = Almost Always
5 = Always

ASSESSMENT RESULTS

Add up your score for each habit. The highest possible score in each category is 50; the higher the score, the better. Please refer to the chart below for interpretation.

ASSESSMENT RESULTS

EAT HEALTHY WITHOUT DIETING	
CONTROL THOSE PORTIONS	
STRENGTH TRAIN	
DO SOME AEROBIC EXERCISE	

SCORE	INTERPRETATION
41-50	EXCELLENT
31-40	GOOD
21-30	NEEDS MODERATE IMPROVEMENT
0-20	NEEDS SIGNIFICANT IMPROVEMENT

CARDIO REFERENCES

AGE	
MAXIMUM HEART RATE (220 - AGE)	
TARGET HEART RATE RANGE FOR MODERATE-INTENSITY ACTIVITY (MAX HR x 0.5 through MAX HR x 0.7)	
TARGET HEART RATE RANGE FOR VIGOROUS-INTENSITY ACTIVITY (MAX HR x 0.7 through MAX HR x 0.85)	

BODY MEASUREMENTS

DATE	
WEIGHT (lbs or kg)	
RIGHT BICEPS (inches or cm)	
WAIST (inches or cm)	
HIPS (inches or cm)	
RIGHT THIGH (inches or cm)	

BLOCK 4

MID-BLOCK MEASUREMENTS

BODY MEASUREMENTS

DATE	
WEIGHT (lbs or kg)	
RIGHT BICEPS (inches or cm)	
WAIST (inches or cm)	
HIPS (inches or cm)	
RIGHT THIGH (inches or cm)	

BLOCK 4

BLOCK 4

MEAL PLANNER

	SUN	MON	TUE	WED	THU	FRI	SAT
WEEK 1 BREAKFAST							
LUNCH							
DINNER							
WEEK 2 BREAKFAST							
LUNCH							
DINNER							
WEEK 3 BREAKFAST							
LUNCH							
DINNER							
WEEK 4 BREAKFAST							
LUNCH							
DINNER							

MEAL PLANNER

BLOCK 4

	SUN	MON	TUE	WED	THU	FRI	SAT
WEEK 5 BREAKFAST / LUNCH / DINNER							
WEEK 6 BREAKFAST / LUNCH / DINNER							
WEEK 7 BREAKFAST / LUNCH / DINNER							
WEEK 8 BREAKFAST / LUNCH / DINNER							

BLOCK 4

MEAL PLANNER

	SUN	MON	TUE	WED	THU	FRI	SAT
WEEK 9 BREAKFAST / LUNCH / DINNER							
WEEK 10 BREAKFAST / LUNCH / DINNER							
WEEK 11 BREAKFAST / LUNCH / DINNER							
WEEK 12 BREAKFAST / LUNCH / DINNER							

BLOCK 4

MY WORKOUT PLAN

12-WEEK CUSTOM WORKOUT SCHEDULE

	SUN	MON	TUE	WED	THU	FRI	SAT
1							
2							
3							
4							
5							
6							
7							
8							
9							
10							
11							
12							

BLOCK 4

BREAD & BUTTER WORKOUTS

UPPER BODY	LOWER BODY	CORE
One Arm Dumbbell Row	Squats	Crunches
Chest Press	Lunges	Leg Raises
Shoulder Press	Dead Lifts	Windshield Wipers
Biceps Curls	Leg Lifts	Mason Twists
Triceps Extensions	Calf Raises	

- Each column is a separate workout. You will only exercise one body section per scheduled workout day.

BLOCK 4

UPPER BODY WORKOUT TRACKER

	WEEK 1	WEEK 2	WEEK 3	WEEK 4	WEEK 5	WEEK 6
ONE ARM ROW	SETS- REPS- WEIGHT-	SETS- REPS- WEIGHT-	SETS- REPS- WEIGHT-	SETS- REPS- WEIGHT-	SETS- REPS- WEIGHT-	SETS- REPS- WEIGHT-
CHEST PRESS	SETS- REPS- WEIGHT-	SETS- REPS- WEIGHT-	SETS- REPS- WEIGHT-	SETS- REPS- WEIGHT-	SETS- REPS- WEIGHT-	SETS- REPS- WEIGHT-
SHOULDER PRESS	SETS- REPS- WEIGHT-	SETS- REPS- WEIGHT-	SETS- REPS- WEIGHT-	SETS- REPS- WEIGHT-	SETS- REPS- WEIGHT-	SETS- REPS- WEIGHT-
BICEPS CURLS	SETS- REPS- WEIGHT-	SETS- REPS- WEIGHT-	SETS- REPS- WEIGHT-	SETS- REPS- WEIGHT-	SETS- REPS- WEIGHT-	SETS- REPS- WEIGHT-
TRICEPS EXTENSIONS	SETS- REPS- WEIGHT-	SETS- REPS- WEIGHT-	SETS- REPS- WEIGHT-	SETS- REPS- WEIGHT-	SETS- REPS- WEIGHT-	SETS- REPS- WEIGHT-

	WEEK 7	WEEK 8	WEEK 9	WEEK 10	WEEK 11	WEEK 12
ONE ARM ROW	SETS- REPS- WEIGHT-	SETS- REPS- WEIGHT-	SETS- REPS- WEIGHT-	SETS- REPS- WEIGHT-	SETS- REPS- WEIGHT-	SETS- REPS- WEIGHT-
CHEST PRESS	SETS- REPS- WEIGHT-	SETS- REPS- WEIGHT-	SETS- REPS- WEIGHT-	SETS- REPS- WEIGHT-	SETS- REPS- WEIGHT-	SETS- REPS- WEIGHT-
SHOULDER PRESS	SETS- REPS- WEIGHT-	SETS- REPS- WEIGHT-	SETS- REPS- WEIGHT-	SETS- REPS- WEIGHT-	SETS- REPS- WEIGHT-	SETS- REPS- WEIGHT-
BICEPS CURLS	SETS- REPS- WEIGHT-	SETS- REPS- WEIGHT-	SETS- REPS- WEIGHT-	SETS- REPS- WEIGHT-	SETS- REPS- WEIGHT-	SETS- REPS- WEIGHT-
TRICEPS EXTENSIONS	SETS- REPS- WEIGHT-	SETS- REPS- WEIGHT-	SETS- REPS- WEIGHT-	SETS- REPS- WEIGHT-	SETS- REPS- WEIGHT-	SETS- REPS- WEIGHT-

BLOCK 4

LOWER BODY WORKOUT TRACKER

	WEEK 1	WEEK 2	WEEK 3	WEEK 4	WEEK 5	WEEK 6
SQUATS	SETS- REPS- WEIGHT-	SETS- REPS- WEIGHT-	SETS- REPS- WEIGHT-	SETS- REPS- WEIGHT-	SETS- REPS- WEIGHT-	SETS- REPS- WEIGHT-
LUNGES	SETS- REPS- WEIGHT-	SETS- REPS- WEIGHT-	SETS- REPS- WEIGHT-	SETS- REPS- WEIGHT-	SETS- REPS- WEIGHT-	SETS- REPS- WEIGHT-
DEAD LIFTS	SETS- REPS- WEIGHT-	SETS- REPS- WEIGHT-	SETS- REPS- WEIGHT-	SETS- REPS- WEIGHT-	SETS- REPS- WEIGHT-	SETS- REPS- WEIGHT-
LEG LIFTS	SETS- REPS- WEIGHT-	SETS- REPS- WEIGHT-	SETS- REPS- WEIGHT-	SETS- REPS- WEIGHT-	SETS- REPS- WEIGHT-	SETS- REPS- WEIGHT-
CALF RAISES	SETS- REPS- WEIGHT-	SETS- REPS- WEIGHT-	SETS- REPS- WEIGHT-	SETS- REPS- WEIGHT-	SETS- REPS- WEIGHT-	SETS- REPS- WEIGHT-

	WEEK 7	WEEK 8	WEEK 9	WEEK 10	WEEK 11	WEEK 12
SQUATS	SETS- REPS- WEIGHT-	SETS- REPS- WEIGHT-	SETS- REPS- WEIGHT-	SETS- REPS- WEIGHT-	SETS- REPS- WEIGHT-	SETS- REPS- WEIGHT-
LUNGES	SETS- REPS- WEIGHT-	SETS- REPS- WEIGHT-	SETS- REPS- WEIGHT-	SETS- REPS- WEIGHT-	SETS- REPS- WEIGHT-	SETS- REPS- WEIGHT-
DEAD LIFTS	SETS- REPS- WEIGHT-	SETS- REPS- WEIGHT-	SETS- REPS- WEIGHT-	SETS- REPS- WEIGHT-	SETS- REPS- WEIGHT-	SETS- REPS- WEIGHT-
LEG LIFTS	SETS- REPS- WEIGHT-	SETS- REPS- WEIGHT-	SETS- REPS- WEIGHT-	SETS- REPS- WEIGHT-	SETS- REPS- WEIGHT-	SETS- REPS- WEIGHT-
CALF RAISES	SETS- REPS- WEIGHT-	SETS- REPS- WEIGHT-	SETS- REPS- WEIGHT-	SETS- REPS- WEIGHT-	SETS- REPS- WEIGHT-	SETS- REPS- WEIGHT-

CORE WORKOUT TRACKER

BLOCK 4

	WEEK 1	WEEK 2	WEEK 3	WEEK 4	WEEK 5	WEEK 6
CRUNCHES	SETS- REPS- WEIGHT-	SETS- REPS- WEIGHT-	SETS- REPS- WEIGHT-	SETS- REPS- WEIGHT-	SETS- REPS- WEIGHT-	SETS- REPS- WEIGHT-
LEG RAISES	SETS- REPS- WEIGHT-	SETS- REPS- WEIGHT-	SETS- REPS- WEIGHT-	SETS- REPS- WEIGHT-	SETS- REPS- WEIGHT-	SETS- REPS- WEIGHT-
WINDSHIELD WIPERS	SETS- REPS- WEIGHT-	SETS- REPS- WEIGHT-	SETS- REPS- WEIGHT-	SETS- REPS- WEIGHT-	SETS- REPS- WEIGHT-	SETS- REPS- WEIGHT-
MASON TWISTS	SETS- REPS- WEIGHT-	SETS- REPS- WEIGHT-	SETS- REPS- WEIGHT-	SETS- REPS- WEIGHT-	SETS- REPS- WEIGHT-	SETS- REPS- WEIGHT-

	WEEK 7	WEEK 8	WEEK 9	WEEK 10	WEEK 11	WEEK 12
CRUNCHES	SETS- REPS- WEIGHT-	SETS- REPS- WEIGHT-	SETS- REPS- WEIGHT-	SETS- REPS- WEIGHT-	SETS- REPS- WEIGHT-	SETS- REPS- WEIGHT-
LEG RAISES	SETS- REPS- WEIGHT-	SETS- REPS- WEIGHT-	SETS- REPS- WEIGHT-	SETS- REPS- WEIGHT-	SETS- REPS- WEIGHT-	SETS- REPS- WEIGHT-
WINDSHIELD WIPERS	SETS- REPS- WEIGHT-	SETS- REPS- WEIGHT-	SETS- REPS- WEIGHT-	SETS- REPS- WEIGHT-	SETS- REPS- WEIGHT-	SETS- REPS- WEIGHT-
MASON TWISTS	SETS- REPS- WEIGHT-	SETS- REPS- WEIGHT-	SETS- REPS- WEIGHT-	SETS- REPS- WEIGHT-	SETS- REPS- WEIGHT-	SETS- REPS- WEIGHT-

NOTES

NOTES

BLOCK 5

START DATE:

END DATE:

HABIT ASSESSMENT

EAT HEALTHY WITHOUT DIETING

1. ____ I eat 2-4 cups of vegetables per day.
2. ____ I eat whole fruits rather than drinking fruit juice.
3. ____ I eat 1-3 cups of fruit per day.
4. ____ I eat a healthy breakfast everyday.
5. ____ I drink at least 8 cups of water a day (64oz).
6. ____ I eat whole wheat bread rather than white bread.
7. ____ I eat whole grain cereals rather than sugary cereals.
8. ____ I eat one or less servings of candy, cake, brownies, cookies, desserts, or similar per day.
9. ____ I eat one or less servings of potato chips, tortilla chips, crackers, or similar snacks per day.
10. ____ I eat a serving of protein with each meal.

SECTION SCORE = _____

CONTROL THOSE PORTIONS

1. ____ At each meal, I dish out a well-balanced plate.
2. ____ I only eat one serving of the meal without going back for seconds.
3. ____ When eating a dessert, unhealthy snack, or candy, I only eat one serving.
4. ____ When I eat protein in a meal (e.g. chicken, beef, fish, eggs, beans, tofu, or other proteins), it is no larger than the size of my fist.
5. ____ When I eat a starchy carbohydrate in a meal (e.g. rice, noodles, pasta, etc.), it is no larger than the size of my fist.
6. ____ When I am given a large portion of food at a restaurant, I eat half and save the other half for a later meal or share the meal with someone.
7. ____ I take my time when eating.
8. ____ I only drink water or low-fat milk with meals.
9. ____ If hungry I eat small healthy snacks in between meals.
10. ____ I avoid using excessive amounts of butter, salad dressing, or condiments.

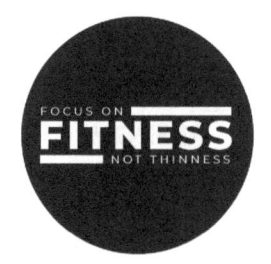

SECTION SCORE = _____

RESPONSE KEY:
0 = Never
1 = Rarely
2 = Sometimes
3 = Often
4 = Almost Always
5 = Always

HABIT ASSESSMENT

STRENGTH TRAIN

1. ____ I do strength training exercises for my arms each week.
2. ____ I do strength training exercises for my legs each week.
3. ____ I work out my core muscles each week.
4. ____ I do exercises using my body weight (e.g. pushups, squats, lunges, plank holds, etc.) as part of my strength training.
5. ____ I use weight lifting equipment (e.g. free weights or weight lifting machines) as part my strength training.
6. ____ I strength train at least two days a week.
7. ____ I give my body time to recover and rebuild by not working out the same body parts two days in a row.
8. ____ I warm up before my strength training exercises.
9. ____ I stretch after each workout to improve my flexibility.
10. ____ I refuel with protein within 30 minutes of finishing a strength training workout.

SECTION SCORE = _____

DO SOME AEROBIC EXERCISE

1. ____ I do some aerobic exercise every week.
2. ____ I take the stairs when I can, rather than the elevator.
3. ____ I park a little farther from store entrances when running errands.
4. ____ When sitting for long periods of time, I intermittently take a few minutes to get up and walk around.
5. ____ I do low-impact aerobic exercises (e.g. ride my bike, elliptical, rower, go swimming, do water aerobics, or similar).
6. ____ I do high-impact aerobic exercises (e.g. brisk walking, jogging, running, jump roping, dancing, playing basketball, soccer, tennis, or similar).
7. ____ I incorporate stretching each time I participate in aerobic exercise.
8. ____ During my aerobic exercise, the intensity is such that I could carry on a conversation rather than gasping for air.
9. ____ I do at least 150 minutes of moderate-intensity or 75 minutes of vigorous-intensity aerobic exercise each week.
10. ____ I strive to stay hydrated during and after my aerobic exercise sessions.

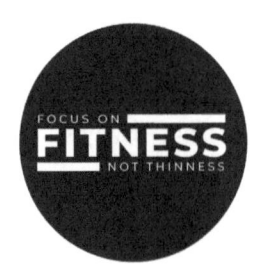

SECTION SCORE = _____

BLOCK 5

RESPONSE KEY:
0 = Never
1 = Rarely
2 = Sometimes
3 = Often
4 = Almost Always
5 = Always

ASSESSMENT RESULTS

Add up your score for each habit. The highest possible score in each category is 50; the higher the score, the better. Please refer to the chart below for interpretation.

ASSESSMENT RESULTS

EAT HEALTHY WITHOUT DIETING	
CONTROL THOSE PORTIONS	
STRENGTH TRAIN	
DO SOME AEROBIC EXERCISE	

SCORE	INTERPRETATION
41-50	EXCELLENT
31-40	GOOD
21-30	NEEDS MODERATE IMPROVEMENT
0-20	NEEDS SIGNIFICANT IMPROVEMENT

CARDIO REFERENCES

AGE	
MAXIMUM HEART RATE (220 - AGE)	
TARGET HEART RATE RANGE FOR MODERATE-INTENSITY ACTIVITY (MAX HR x 0.5 through MAX HR x 0.7)	
TARGET HEART RATE RANGE FOR VIGOROUS-INTENSITY ACTIVITY (MAX HR x 0.7 through MAX HR x 0.85)	

BODY MEASUREMENTS

DATE	
WEIGHT (lbs or kg)	
RIGHT BICEPS (inches or cm)	
WAIST (inches or cm)	
HIPS (inches or cm)	
RIGHT THIGH (inches or cm)	

MID-BLOCK MEASUREMENTS

BODY MEASUREMENTS

DATE	
WEIGHT (lbs or kg)	
RIGHT BICEPS (inches or cm)	
WAIST (inches or cm)	
HIPS (inches or cm)	
RIGHT THIGH (inches or cm)	

BLOCK 5

BLOCK 5

MEAL PLANNER

	SUN	MON	TUE	WED	THU	FRI	SAT
WEEK 1 BREAKFAST							
LUNCH							
DINNER							
WEEK 2 BREAKFAST							
LUNCH							
DINNER							
WEEK 3 BREAKFAST							
LUNCH							
DINNER							
WEEK 4 BREAKFAST							
LUNCH							
DINNER							

MEAL PLANNER

BLOCK 5

	SUN	MON	TUE	WED	THU	FRI	SAT
WEEK 5 BREAKFAST / LUNCH / DINNER							
WEEK 6 BREAKFAST / LUNCH / DINNER							
WEEK 7 BREAKFAST / LUNCH / DINNER							
WEEK 8 BREAKFAST / LUNCH / DINNER							

BLOCK 5

MEAL PLANNER

	SUN	MON	TUE	WED	THU	FRI	SAT
WEEK 9 BREAKFAST / LUNCH / DINNER							
WEEK 10 BREAKFAST / LUNCH / DINNER							
WEEK 11 BREAKFAST / LUNCH / DINNER							
WEEK 12 BREAKFAST / LUNCH / DINNER							

MY WORKOUT PLAN

12-WEEK CUSTOM WORKOUT SCHEDULE

BLOCK 5

	SUN	MON	TUE	WED	THU	FRI	SAT
1							
2							
3							
4							
5							
6							
7							
8							
9							
10							
11							
12							

BLOCK 5

BREAD & BUTTER WORKOUTS

UPPER BODY

LOWER BODY

CORE

Upper Body	Lower Body	Core
One Arm Dumbbell Row	Squats	Crunches
Chest Press	Lunges	Leg Raises
Shoulder Press	Dead Lifts	Windshield Wipers
Biceps Curls	Leg Lifts	Mason Twists
Triceps Extensions	Calf Raises	

- Each column is a separate workout. You will only exercise one body section per scheduled workout day.

UPPER BODY WORKOUT TRACKER

BLOCK 5

	WEEK 1	WEEK 2	WEEK 3	WEEK 4	WEEK 5	WEEK 6
ONE ARM ROW	SETS- REPS- WEIGHT-	SETS- REPS- WEIGHT-	SETS- REPS- WEIGHT-	SETS- REPS- WEIGHT-	SETS- REPS- WEIGHT-	SETS- REPS- WEIGHT-
CHEST PRESS	SETS- REPS- WEIGHT-	SETS- REPS- WEIGHT-	SETS- REPS- WEIGHT-	SETS- REPS- WEIGHT-	SETS- REPS- WEIGHT-	SETS- REPS- WEIGHT-
SHOULDER PRESS	SETS- REPS- WEIGHT-	SETS- REPS- WEIGHT-	SETS- REPS- WEIGHT-	SETS- REPS- WEIGHT-	SETS- REPS- WEIGHT-	SETS- REPS- WEIGHT-
BICEPS CURLS	SETS- REPS- WEIGHT-	SETS- REPS- WEIGHT-	SETS- REPS- WEIGHT-	SETS- REPS- WEIGHT-	SETS- REPS- WEIGHT-	SETS- REPS- WEIGHT-
TRICEPS EXTENSIONS	SETS- REPS- WEIGHT-	SETS- REPS- WEIGHT-	SETS- REPS- WEIGHT-	SETS- REPS- WEIGHT-	SETS- REPS- WEIGHT-	SETS- REPS- WEIGHT-

	WEEK 7	WEEK 8	WEEK 9	WEEK 10	WEEK 11	WEEK 12
ONE ARM ROW	SETS- REPS- WEIGHT-	SETS- REPS- WEIGHT-	SETS- REPS- WEIGHT-	SETS- REPS- WEIGHT-	SETS- REPS- WEIGHT-	SETS- REPS- WEIGHT-
CHEST PRESS	SETS- REPS- WEIGHT-	SETS- REPS- WEIGHT-	SETS- REPS- WEIGHT-	SETS- REPS- WEIGHT-	SETS- REPS- WEIGHT-	SETS- REPS- WEIGHT-
SHOULDER PRESS	SETS- REPS- WEIGHT-	SETS- REPS- WEIGHT-	SETS- REPS- WEIGHT-	SETS- REPS- WEIGHT-	SETS- REPS- WEIGHT-	SETS- REPS- WEIGHT-
BICEPS CURLS	SETS- REPS- WEIGHT-	SETS- REPS- WEIGHT-	SETS- REPS- WEIGHT-	SETS- REPS- WEIGHT-	SETS- REPS- WEIGHT-	SETS- REPS- WEIGHT-
TRICEPS EXTENSIONS	SETS- REPS- WEIGHT-	SETS- REPS- WEIGHT-	SETS- REPS- WEIGHT-	SETS- REPS- WEIGHT-	SETS- REPS- WEIGHT-	SETS- REPS- WEIGHT-

BLOCK 5

LOWER BODY WORKOUT TRACKER

	WEEK 1	WEEK 2	WEEK 3	WEEK 4	WEEK 5	WEEK 6
SQUATS	SETS- REPS- WEIGHT-	SETS- REPS- WEIGHT-	SETS- REPS- WEIGHT-	SETS- REPS- WEIGHT-	SETS- REPS- WEIGHT-	SETS- REPS- WEIGHT-
LUNGES	SETS- REPS- WEIGHT-	SETS- REPS- WEIGHT-	SETS- REPS- WEIGHT-	SETS- REPS- WEIGHT-	SETS- REPS- WEIGHT-	SETS- REPS- WEIGHT-
DEAD LIFTS	SETS- REPS- WEIGHT-	SETS- REPS- WEIGHT-	SETS- REPS- WEIGHT-	SETS- REPS- WEIGHT-	SETS- REPS- WEIGHT-	SETS- REPS- WEIGHT-
LEG LIFTS	SETS- REPS- WEIGHT-	SETS- REPS- WEIGHT-	SETS- REPS- WEIGHT-	SETS- REPS- WEIGHT-	SETS- REPS- WEIGHT-	SETS- REPS- WEIGHT-
CALF RAISES	SETS- REPS- WEIGHT-	SETS- REPS- WEIGHT-	SETS- REPS- WEIGHT-	SETS- REPS- WEIGHT-	SETS- REPS- WEIGHT-	SETS- REPS- WEIGHT-

	WEEK 7	WEEK 8	WEEK 9	WEEK 10	WEEK 11	WEEK 12
SQUATS	SETS- REPS- WEIGHT-	SETS- REPS- WEIGHT-	SETS- REPS- WEIGHT-	SETS- REPS- WEIGHT-	SETS- REPS- WEIGHT-	SETS- REPS- WEIGHT-
LUNGES	SETS- REPS- WEIGHT-	SETS- REPS- WEIGHT-	SETS- REPS- WEIGHT-	SETS- REPS- WEIGHT-	SETS- REPS- WEIGHT-	SETS- REPS- WEIGHT-
DEAD LIFTS	SETS- REPS- WEIGHT-	SETS- REPS- WEIGHT-	SETS- REPS- WEIGHT-	SETS- REPS- WEIGHT-	SETS- REPS- WEIGHT-	SETS- REPS- WEIGHT-
LEG LIFTS	SETS- REPS- WEIGHT-	SETS- REPS- WEIGHT-	SETS- REPS- WEIGHT-	SETS- REPS- WEIGHT-	SETS- REPS- WEIGHT-	SETS- REPS- WEIGHT-
CALF RAISES	SETS- REPS- WEIGHT-	SETS- REPS- WEIGHT-	SETS- REPS- WEIGHT-	SETS- REPS- WEIGHT-	SETS- REPS- WEIGHT-	SETS- REPS- WEIGHT-

CORE WORKOUT TRACKER

BLOCK 5

	WEEK 1	WEEK 2	WEEK 3	WEEK 4	WEEK 5	WEEK 6
CRUNCHES	SETS- REPS- WEIGHT-	SETS- REPS- WEIGHT-	SETS- REPS- WEIGHT-	SETS- REPS- WEIGHT-	SETS- REPS- WEIGHT-	SETS- REPS- WEIGHT-
LEG RAISES	SETS- REPS- WEIGHT-	SETS- REPS- WEIGHT-	SETS- REPS- WEIGHT-	SETS- REPS- WEIGHT-	SETS- REPS- WEIGHT-	SETS- REPS- WEIGHT-
WINDSHIELD WIPERS	SETS- REPS- WEIGHT-	SETS- REPS- WEIGHT-	SETS- REPS- WEIGHT-	SETS- REPS- WEIGHT-	SETS- REPS- WEIGHT-	SETS- REPS- WEIGHT-
MASON TWISTS	SETS- REPS- WEIGHT-	SETS- REPS- WEIGHT-	SETS- REPS- WEIGHT-	SETS- REPS- WEIGHT-	SETS- REPS- WEIGHT-	SETS- REPS- WEIGHT-

	WEEK 7	WEEK 8	WEEK 9	WEEK 10	WEEK 11	WEEK 12
CRUNCHES	SETS- REPS- WEIGHT-	SETS- REPS- WEIGHT-	SETS- REPS- WEIGHT-	SETS- REPS- WEIGHT-	SETS- REPS- WEIGHT-	SETS- REPS- WEIGHT-
LEG RAISES	SETS- REPS- WEIGHT-	SETS- REPS- WEIGHT-	SETS- REPS- WEIGHT-	SETS- REPS- WEIGHT-	SETS- REPS- WEIGHT-	SETS- REPS- WEIGHT-
WINDSHIELD WIPERS	SETS- REPS- WEIGHT-	SETS- REPS- WEIGHT-	SETS- REPS- WEIGHT-	SETS- REPS- WEIGHT-	SETS- REPS- WEIGHT-	SETS- REPS- WEIGHT-
MASON TWISTS	SETS- REPS- WEIGHT-	SETS- REPS- WEIGHT-	SETS- REPS- WEIGHT-	SETS- REPS- WEIGHT-	SETS- REPS- WEIGHT-	SETS- REPS- WEIGHT-

NOTES

NOTES

NOTES

NOTES

NOTES

NOTES

Made in United States
Troutdale, OR
06/12/2025